THE
CLEAR SKIN
DIET

THE
CLEAR SKIN
DIET

HOW TO DEFEAT ACNE AND ENJOY HEALTHY SKIN

Alan C. Logan, ND, FRSH   Valori Treloar MD, CNS, FAAD

CUMBERLAND HOUSE

THE CLEAR SKIN DIET

PUBLISHED BY CUMBERLAND HOUSE PUBLISHING, AN IMPRINT OF SOURCEBOOKS, INC.

P.O. Box 4410

Naperville, IL 60567-4410

www.sourcebooks.com

Cover design: Gore Studio, Inc.

Library of Congress Cataloging-in-Publication Data
Logan, Alan C.
  The Clear skin diet : how to defeat acne and enjoy healthy skin / Alan C. Logan, Valori Treloar.
      p. cm.
  Includes bibliographical references and index.
  1. Acne,Treatment. 2. Acne—Diet therapy. 3. Acne—Nutritional aspects. I. Treloar, Valori, 1953– II. Title.
  RL131.L64 2007
  616.5'3—dc22

                                                                                    2007024741

Printed in the United States of America
SB 11

This book is dedicated to the medical professionals and scientists who continue to think outside the box. Thanks for demonstrating that the only myth concerning acne and diet is that which states there is no connection between the two.

CONTENTS

Foreword

It's a serious compliment to be asked to write a foreword. The opportunity doesn't come along often, and in addition to thanking Val Treloar and Alan Logan for the opportunity, I want to thank a few patients who set me to thinking and started this all rolling around in my head. One of the first was a sixty-one-year-old gent whose back was a veritable moonscape of active acne and who had eaten a pint of ice cream daily for the previous half century. Another was the "always spotty" Scottish lass, an identical twin whose clear-skinned sister couldn't bear drinking whole milk and drank only minimal amounts of the partially skimmed "bottom of the milk bottle" from the days before homogenized milk. My patient loved milk; indeed she would scoop the cream from the top when she could. More recent was the delightful twenty-eight-year-old miss with previously flawless skin who wished to open a deli so spent several months traveling Europe learning about, and consuming, the best cheeses of several countries. She presented with nodulocystic acne from ear to ear along her jaw line, but she made the diagnosis herself during my opening search for the trigger. "Omigod," she said, "it's the cheese."

All of this led me eventually to approach, with considerable trepidation, the high priest of nutritional epidemiological studies, Dr. Walter Willett, the Fredrick John Stare Professor of Epidemiology and Nutrition, Department of Nutrition, Harvard School of Public Health.

I think I detected some incredulity during our initial meeting, but for reasons we've never discussed, he must have wondered if there was something to it because he assigned Clement Adebamowo, a postdoctoral fellow, to the work. After a lot of heavy lifting, Clement had his Sc.D., I had my thirty-year-old question answered, and the association between milk and acne was proven.

The word association is important because we are still are puzzling over the molecular mechanisms involved, but the original work has led further, and following my presentation on the subject to the Massachusetts Academy of Dermatology a few years ago, Val Treloar quietly presented herself and we got to talking . . . and talking . . . and talking. I found that Val, partly because of her additional training but more out of a deep and abiding interest, has an encyclopedic knowledge of the relationship of foods to our most important hormonal and inflammatory processes. This extends far and away beyond my grasp and, as she points out, far beyond what is taught to (or learned by) today's (and yesterday's) medical students.

What she and Dr. Logan have set out for us here is the most thorough review of the subject ever undertaken. It covers the ground from naturopathy through holistic medicine, from junk food through healthy nutrition, from classic medical dermatology and integrative medicine through today's pharma-driven dermatology and what we think is "scientific" dermatology, and ties it all in to our relationship with the foods we eat. It takes us from the days we followed Osler's teaching and listened to our patients, right up to the present where, if it isn't on a "drop-down" menu sitting in front of a "physician extender," an important part of the history will be missed entirely.

Importantly, this book also reminds us of the days when physicians assimilated information from their patients, and that process led to concepts of disease. Who today would do what Pasadena dermatologist Jerome Fisher did thirty years ago: sit down and take a detailed dietary history from more than a thousand consecutive acne patients? And guess what? Those early observers were in many instances remarkably perspicacious—and watching the authors draw those links is just one great reason to read this book.

Another reason is to learn more about the relationship between your food and your health than you would have thought possible. This is not just about acne and food; this is about life.

This book will open your eyes, I promise; and your mind, I hope.

BILL DANBY, MD, FRCP(C)
SECTION OF DERMATOLOGY, DEPARTMENT OF MEDICINE
DARTMOUTH UNIVERSITY

Acknowledgements

Alan writes . . .

I am deeply indebted to Dr. Valori Treloar for opening the door and agreeing to collaborate on this project. Immediately it became very clear that Valori is a walking encyclopedia and a very special dermatologist who prioritizes the needs of her patients. Valori's training, clinical experience, nutritional expertise, and integrative approach proved invaluable. I learned so much from Valori as she carefully sculpted *The Clear Skin Diet*.

A special thanks to two of the nation's most talented illustrators—Certified Medical Illustrator Marcia Hartsock of the Medical Art Company and Stan Yan of Squidworks for their wonderful contributions to this text. I am grateful to Valorie et al. from the Westchester Public Library System, who turned over every stone to secure many articles from medical and scientific journals, including our prized copy of the 1942 text *Fundamentals of Medical Dermatology*. Thanks to my good friends and colleagues in Toronto for all your support.

Thanks to my wife Yoshiko for your love and support through this writing, and for being the best mom in the world to our boy Kaz. Thanks also for the translation of the Japanese journal articles, and for being the tour guide to the particulars of the traditional Japanese diet!

Valori writes . . .

I am grateful to my coauthor Alan Logan, who did the lion's share of writing this book, for allowing me to tinker with it and selfishly mold it into a tool that suited my needs and those of my patients. His generosity and selflessness astonish me still.

I thank my courageous patients who strive to understand their diseases and embrace life changes in order to be healthier. I am lucky to be able to work with you and learn with you.

Ross Sharp and Elizabeth Fitzpayne, the librarians at Newton-Wellesley Hospital and the Massachusetts Medical Society, helped me far more than they should have. Thanks for stretching the rules a bit. Lincoln Street Coffee was my second office and fueled many pages of writing with excellent lattes.

Nothing can compare to the blessing of a nutty, loving family. My husband and kids, in particular, must be credited for their stoic patience.

Introduction

The idea of a diet to promote clear, healthy skin, free of acne, is certainly not a new one. Some seventy years ago, nutrition and lifestyle were at the forefront of dermatological education and care. The primary textbook of the day, *Fundamentals of Medical Dermatology* (1942), placed great emphasis on quality nutrition, a healthy intestinal tract, restful sleep, minimization of stress, and physical activity. However, by the early 1970s, with the explosion of pharmaceutical-driven science, and with the assistance of two poorly designed chocolate studies (which we will discuss), diet and lifestyle fell out of favor. The official position of most dermatological authorities was that there was no connection between diet/lifestyle and acne. For the next thirty years, diet was dismissed from dermatological training, relegated to "myth" status, leading to patients being dismissed when they brought up ideas that diet might be aggravating their acne.

Today we are excited to witness a new history being written in the annals of dermatological care—the winds of change have swept in, taking the form of exciting new research publications. The new research validates what patients and old-school dermatology training were saying—diet and lifestyle matter! In *The Clear Skin Diet* we will transport you through this history and update you on the latest research regarding diet, lifestyle, and acne.

The starting point is the acne process itself, its causes, presentation, and conventional treatment. The backdrop to our approach is, of course, the sad reality of the typical North American diet with its current excesses and nutritional voids. In chapter 2 we will carry you through the modern history of nutritional medicine and highlight the poor scientific rationale that became the reason why you have probably been told or read that there is no connection between diet and acne. Moving forward through chapter 3, we will explain why anti-inflammatory and antioxidant-rich foods can dampen the acne process. In particular, we will focus on the therapeutic potential of omega-3 fatty acids.

In recent years, scientists have discovered that various aspects of the diet can have a significant effect in the elevation or reduction of the very hormones that ultimately drive acne. In chapter 4 we will discuss the key elements that can promote clear skin through hormonal influences. In following the advice of dermatologists practicing seventy years ago, we will revive the focus on and value of intestinal health for clear skin. The major difference is that there have been major advances in science documenting the role of gut bacteria in promoting health, including aspects of health far removed from the reaches of the intestinal tract—the skin, it turns out, is no exception. Stress has recently been shown to be an acne promoter, and we have provided in-depth discussions on this connection. In particular, we focus on utilizing the approaches of the discipline of mind-body medicine in prevention and promotion of clear skin.

We acknowledge that the contents of *The Clear Skin Diet* are not superficial, and some of the discussion can have considerable depth. We believe that this allows for completeness and a true understanding of the mechanisms by which diet and lifestyle can influence the pathways of acne. Wherever possible, we have made every effort to simplify this information for ease of understanding and, ultimately, practical application. This, we hope, will become very clear in the Action Plan for the Clear Skin Diet—a synthesis of the text into need-to-know information, the daily game plan for a clear skin lifestyle. *Lifestyle* is the key word. Diet, as you will see, is but one aspect of the four pillars (sleep, relaxation response, exercise, and diet) that make up the Action Plan.

We hope that the combined authorship of a complementary medicine provider and a conventionally trained dermatologist translates well into a complete action plan for your clear skin. We have come from different medical training backgrounds, yet our experiences and research have converged on the common ground of nutrition and lifestyle factors in illness. Both of us are conservative in our approach, and we underscore that the four-part Action Plan diet/lifestyle we advocate is not a substitute for appropriate dermatological evaluation and care. We view our Action Plan as well suited to be an adjunct to the primary interventions of skilled dermatologists. It is also important to point out that diet and lifestyle changes may not work well for everyone, particularly in cases of severe acne. Share your intentions with your doctor, and always disclose your use of dietary supplements. It may be helpful to share your copy of *The Clear Skin Diet* with your dermatologist—he or she, like you, may be pleasantly surprised by the outcome of a complete, integrative approach.

Your acne is considered SEVERE if you have:

1. More than 10–15 red bumps or pustules (red bumps with pus) on the face, chest, and/or back
2. Acne nodules (red bumps bigger than about ⅓ inch in diameter, or the size of a cranberry
3. Pitted or bumpy scars from acne

If your acne falls into one or more of these categories, the guidelines in this book are likely to improve your health, but may not be enough to treat your acne. Please make an appointment with a dermatologist. The Action Plan for Clear Skin will not interfere with conventional acne treatment. You may use it in conjunction with your doctor's program.

We are excited to see the dawning of a new era in dermatology. After a long hiatus, diet and lifestyle are back in the fold again. We have much respect and appreciation for the small group of international dermatologists and researchers who kept the torch alive over the years. We also appreciate the efforts of those who have refused to let the old chocolate studies impede further evaluation of the acne-diet connection. Based on the emerging research, we anticipate that dermatologists will soon reclaim their rightful place as nutrition and lifestyle experts through proper training in residency and continuing education. The truth is that for many young patients, dermatologists are often the first doctors to be queried on the topic of nutrition. This represents a wonderful opportunity for shared discussion and education on diet and lifestyle—proper instruction may invoke changes that not only have the potential to promote clear skin, but also to help establish diet and lifestyle habits that promote good health for life.

Yours in Health!

ALAN C. LOGAN, ND, FRSH   VALORI TRELOAR, MD, CNS, FAAD
ANXIETY CENTER AT WHITE
PLAINS HOSPITAL   INTEGRATIVE DERMATOLOGY
WHITE PLAINS, NY   NEWTON, MA
WWW.DRLOGAN.COM   WWW.INTEGRATIVEDERM.COM

THE
CLEAR SKIN
DIET

1

ACNE AND NUTRITIONAL REALITIES

ACNE IS A CHRONIC SKIN condition that is experienced, to one degree or another, by the majority of those living in Western nations. While acne may be thought of as a self-limiting condition that is outgrown by the twentieth birthday, research indicates otherwise. There has been a significant increase in acne through all ages in the last half century, and many adults are now experiencing acne for the first time. At the dawning of the new millennium, an editorial in the prestigious dermatology journal *Cutis* (2001) referred to adult acne as a "worldwide epidemic." There are now approximately twenty million adults diagnosed with acne in North America, with millions more who do not seek medical care.

In a recent study published in the *British Journal of Dermatology* (2005), researchers examined the changing rates of acne among university students spanning the latter decades of the twentieth century. The results showed that acne rates have indeed significantly increased among students since 1948. As highlighted in a recent issue of *U.S. News and World Report* (November 14, 2005), aptly titled "Oh, no! Not at my age!" the research also shows that more and more adults are dealing with acne. The average age of patients in acne clinics has increased from twenty years old in 1984 to twenty-six years old in 1994. Millions of adults, and women in particular, many of whom may have escaped teenage acne, are living with new outbreaks. Since conventional wisdom suggests that acne is very much a genetically dictated condition, how could there be a rise in acne rates? What's happening here?

The researchers from the University of Bristol, U.K., who uncovered the rise in acne among university students stated, "We suggest that environmental exposure may underlie this, as changes in the prevalence of germline genetic variants are very unlikely to occur in such a short time period." In other words, the genetic pool of the students who attended university was pretty much the same at both ends of the twenty-year evaluation, so there must be something else going on—that something else is most likely an environmental variable that can easily change in the course of twenty years. The most obvious candidates among environmental exposures that have varied in the last half century are lifestyle, stressors, and, yes, diet. These variables are known to influence the genes we have, so, despite genetic susceptibilities, the onset of or course of a medical condition is influenced by such factors as stress and nutrition. This is especially true for chronic medical conditions where there are multiple factors involved—cardiovascular disease, obesity, diabetes, and neurodegenerative diseases such as Alzheimer's are well-known examples. Acne, as we will discuss, is a prime example of a complex, chronic medical condition that is influenced by many factors.

The research cited throughout this book will make it painfully obvious that the only myth surrounding acne and diet is that which states there is no relationship between the two—sadly, many doctors hold onto strong beliefs, and even in the face of new evidence, they can't let them go. Sometimes vision is clouded by the vested interest in patented prescription skin creams and pills, but mostly it's due to lack of attention paid to the advances of nutritional medicine. The two oft-cited studies conducted almost forty years ago on an acne-diet connection, viewed through modern research filters, are so full of design holes it would make a Swiss cheese maker proud. The studies both concluded that there is no connection between chocolate and other high-fat foods and acne. Until recently, there was little further attention paid to the subject of diet and acne, and generations of dermatologists have grown up believing for the most part that there is no relationship between the two.

Before we begin trolling the acne-nutrition-lifestyle relationships, we must underscore that although the research shows that nutritional influences have been unfairly dismissed, they are not everything in acne. Dietary changes may not help everyone to the same degree, and it is also true that nutritional interventions are certainly not a substitute for appropriate dermatological care. The Clear Skin Diet is not an overly restrictive diet—it is, however, one that is based entirely on the inclusion of well-documented healthy eating habits—nutritional inclusions that are known to have numerous collateral benefits to general health. The only restrictive portion of the Clear Skin Diet is related to foods that may be fueling acne and compromising its healing process—we place limits on the same types of foods and beverages that have been consistently tied to long-term health problems such as cardiovascular disease, obesity, and diabetes. Our plan is not a "detox" diet, or other such vague, overhyped approach with no scientific evidence related to acne. It is not a seven-day plan, a fourteen-day plan, or any other such time-oriented approach. It is a lifestyle for the promotion of healthy eating habits and stress reduction; it is a lifestyle for daily, weekly, monthly, and annual use, one that will help keep acne at bay and support the overall health of your mind and body.

Marketing Magicians

Each year there are upwards of eight million visits to office-based physicians where acne is the diagnosis or reason for the visit. Countless more adults and teens with acne never see a dermatologist and rely upon overpaid Hollywood celebrities to direct them to the testimonial-driven goods—you know, the cable-TV products—which, by the way, contain active ingredients that have been readily available over-the-counter in most drugstores for years. Millions around the globe pick up the phone and fork over the big bucks for products with limited research. It seems in every country we visit overseas, from Tokyo, Japan, to Belfast, Northern Ireland, we see the usual cast of American celebs hawking the same branded acne products on late-night TV. The various over-the-counter products account for more than $100 million per year in sales, and the overall annual cost of health care related to the treatment of acne exceeds $1 billion in the

United States alone. While these numbers may seem staggering, the sheer distress of acne leads to desperation. The marketing spin doctors are well aware that most patients are willing to spend their last nickel on the treatment of acne. Despite not being in and of itself a life-threatening condition, acne can severely damage quality of life—in fact, research shows that the emotional fallout from having acne can be worse than that related to asthma or even epilepsy. Researchers reported in the *British Journal of Dermatology* (1999) that 62 percent of adults with acne experience anxiety and/or depression, sometimes even clinical levels thereof, and the psychological damage can persist for years.

Pathology and Current Treatments

Before we explore the issues of diet and acne in the following chapters, let's look first at acne itself, the causes and treatments. While there are a number of skin conditions that include the word *acne* in the description (e.g., acne rosacea), the focus of this text is on the classic, most common, and well-known form—acne vulgaris. We generally consider the "typical" acne patient to be a teen; however, the age range includes newborns, the elderly, and every age in between. Acne includes not only a range of different kinds of visible lesions (comedones, papules, pustules, and nodules, which we will discuss); the disease itself can vary along a wide spectrum from very mild to extremely severe. Acne is unquestionably a highly variable disease. *The Clear Skin Diet* delves deeply into the subject of acne, drawing on the latest complex developments in dermatology and the science behind the nutritional/lifestyle influences, which, in the end, provides for a more complete picture and fills in some of the holes that currently exist in this emerging area of nutritional medicine.

Acne is described as a disease of the "pilosebaceous units" of the skin—medical jargon for the small oil-producing areas and tiny hairs that make up your pores. At this point we need you to say "pilosebaceous unit" ten times quickly so that it becomes a familiar term, again, referring to the area underlying each pore on the surface of your skin. The actual canal under the pore is referred to as the follicle, and therein resides a tiny hair and an oil gland. The oil gland is known medically as the sebaceous gland, and its job is to secrete an oily substance called sebum. Old dermatology textbooks also referred to the sebaceous gland as the "fat gland." Because the oil-producing cells in the sebaceous gland are continuously being replaced by new growth at the base of the glands, sebum is really a combination of fat and the debris of dead fat-producing cells. The sebum is dumped on the hairs inside the follicles and is brought up to the surface of the skin along the hair shaft. Under normal circumstances, things work according to plan, and the oil gland helps remove old skin cells and serves to keep the skin well lubricated.

There are four major problems in the pilosebaceous unit when it comes to acne:

1. Hyperplasia of the oil-producing sebaceous gland—medical jargon for increased turnover/production of cells of the gland. In practical terms, this translates into excessive sebum production.

2. Hyperkeratinization of the hair follicle—again, increased turnover/production of the cells, but this time it is those cells lining the follicle walls. These cells fail to loosen so they don't fall away from the follicle wall. In practical terms, this translates into obstruction or clogging of the canal.

3. Proliferation and colonization of Propionibacterium acnes—put simply, this normal bacterial resident of the follicle overgrows. While acne can occur in the absence of P. acnes bacteria, research has shown that it contributes to blockage and provokes an immune system response that causes inflammation. In addition, 68 percent of acne papules contain a yeast called Malassezia that adds even more irritants.

4. As a result of major problems 1–3 listed above, the follicle itself can rupture and leak bacteria, fats, and other gunk into the dermis, the area of skin cells surrounding the follicle—and significant inflammation and oxidative stress (free-radical generation) can result.

These steps lead to open comedones (blackheads) and the even more dreaded closed comedones (whiteheads). Throw in the inflammatory process, and you end up with larger red bumps (papules) and those that have the yellowish pus (pustules) on display. When the inflammation occurs just a little bit deeper in the skin, it takes the form of large red, painful, and firm nodular acne blemishes. Sometimes pitted scars persist after the lesions heal. Hormones are a major player, especially in kicking off the process at step one in the sebaceous gland and the accumulation of follicle lining cells. New research indicates that chemicals derived from the nervous system can also innervate the sebaceous gland and promote the production of sebum. Substance P, most well-known as a chemical that promotes pain in the human body, is a nervous system chemical recently noted to promote sebum production. Interestingly, substance P may also be influencing the depression and anxiety that are often part and parcel of acne. As we will discuss, dietary quality can influence the hormones and nervous system chemicals responsible for sebaceous gland as well as follicle structure and function. Dietary fats and foods that cause an elevation in insulin can also affect sebum and follicle cell production. A variety of foods and the nutrients within them can also exert significant anti-inflammatory and antioxidant properties that can dampen the cascade involved in acne. In addition, the dietary and supplemental administration of certain beneficial bacteria that normally reside in the gastrointestinal tract can have a marked impact on lowering inflammation and decreasing oxidative stress throughout the body. Obviously we have lots to discuss; however, before doing so, here are the mainstream approaches.

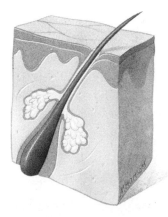

The Normal Hair Follicle—All is well; the sebaceous glands are of normal size, and the follicle walls are shedding cells at a normal rate.

The Open Comedo—Trouble is brewing, and the blackhead has formed due to the failure of the cells to shed, causing buildup and improper expulsion of cells. A mixture of cells, fat, and other gunk, the blackhead is not darkly colored from dirt—collection of the skin pigment melanin reacting with oxygen provides the color.

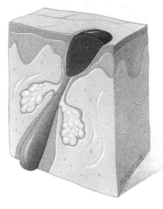

The Closed Comedo—This is the classic whitehead, and it is caused by the same buildup of retained cells and sebum—the only difference is that because it is closed and unopened to the surface, the appearance remains white because there is no reaction with melanin in the absence of air exposure.

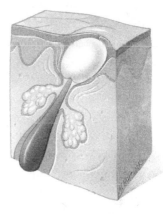

Acne-Promoting Medications

Most Common	Least Common
anabolic steroids (testosterone, danazol)	azathioprine
	cyclosporine
bromides	disulfiram (Antabuse)
corticosteriods (prednisone)	phenobarbitol
corticotropin	quinidine
isoniazid	tetracycline
lithium	excess B vitamins—(B1, B6, B12)
phenytoin	
DHEA	

The Papule—Worse trouble here; the follicle can no longer contain the contents that are building up with nowhere to go. Local immune reaction causes the characteristic red bump on the skin surface, which can be up to half a centimeter in diameter.

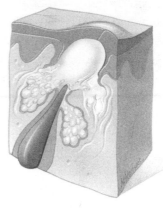

The Pustule—The dam has burst and things are getting out of hand. The blockage has caused a considerable spillover into the surrounding area beyond the follicle. Now the whole package also contains a large collection of white blood cells and bacteria that combine to provide the yellow pus color on the surface. Inflammation is significant and free-radical damage is apparent. If the top seals over, an improper healing process can lead to a walled-off cyst and an increased risk of scarring.

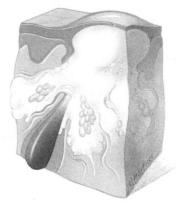

Treatment

The sales of acne medications bypassed the one billion dollar mark in 1999 and have risen steadily since then. Over-the-counter preparations sold in department stores, supermarkets, and drugstores are gaining ground quickly with over $800 million in global sales as of 2005. These numbers speak volumes about the sense of suffering and desperation of acne patients of all ages. The conventional treatment of acne is usually dictated by its severity, with topical preparations being the first choice in more mild cases, while medications that work from the inside out are generally reserved for moderate to severe cases. Heading to the local drugstore or calling an 800 number after being mesmerized by a celebrity hawking a product will generally put you in the direction of three active ingredients available without a prescription.

OVER-THE-COUNTER TOPICALS

1. Benzoyl Peroxide Creams, Cleansers, or Gels—Despite being on the market for years, the precise mechanisms by which BP can, in some people, improve mild-to-moderate acne remains something of a mystery. It is known that BP has an antibacterial effect against P. acnes, so that may be one mechanism, and an anti-inflammatory effect has also been postulated. It certainly dries out the skin and can cause flaking; however, according to a large review in the journal Drugs (2004), it does not have an effect on the oil-producing sebaceous gland, nor does it affect the production of cells lining the pilosebaceous unit. It does cause free-radical damage, and some suggest that this is a good thing because it causes damage to and breaks up the comedo, the plug of dead skin and fat that blocks the follicle. BP may also create an oxygen-rich environment that, in turn, inhibits the growth of P. acnes. It is the primary active ingredient in the overhyped cable-TV infomercials.

2. Salicylic Acid Pads, Gels, Lotions, or Cleansers—These formulations usually have concentrations of SA that vary between 0.5 and 2 percent. SA can prevent the formation of the comedo by exfoliating the cells that line the follicle, and there are some encouraging placebo-controlled studies that support efficacy. Some head-to-head studies show SA to be more effective than benzoyl peroxide.

3. Glycolic Acid Creams, Peels, Lotions, Cleansers—Glycolic acid also works as an exfoliant to clear out the follicle before the formation of a comedo. While studies using 35–70 percent glycolic acid do show benefit in acne, little is known about the 6 percent glycolic acid solutions promoted by celebrities on late-night cable TV. Sadly, there is no research published on the scientific

How Effective Is Proactiv?

Survey questions posed to study subjects with averages from patient assessment scores with both therapies on the 10-point scale used (Burkhart et al., International Journal of Dermatology 2007, 46, 89–93. Reprinted with permission of Blackwell Synergy)

1. How did the treatment perform in reducing the severity of your acne? (1, no improvement; 10, fabulous improvement)
   Proactiv Solution, 4.3; benzoyl peroxide–allylamine, 7.0
2. How did the treatment perform in reducing the number of acne lesions? (1, no improvement; 10, did extremely well)
   Proactiv Solution, 4.3; benzoyl peroxide–allylamine, 7.1
3. How did the treatment perform in reducing the amount of redness of acne? (1, no improvement; 10, did extremely well)
   Proactiv Solution, 4.3; benzoyl peroxide–allylamine, 5.6
4. How easy was the acne treatment to do every day? (1, very difficult; 10, very easy)
   Proactiv Solution, 7.5; benzoyl peroxide–allylamine, 7.9
5. Does your skin feel softer to you at the completion of the study? (1, much tougher; 5, same as originally; 10, much softer)
   Proactiv Solution, 5.8; benzoyl peroxide–allylamine, 6.1
6. Does your skin feel smoother to you at the completion of the study? (1, much rougher; 5, same as originally; 10, much smoother)
   Proactiv Solution, 5.5; benzoyl peroxide–allylamine, 6.6
7. Did the product you used seem to prevent breakouts? (1, not at all; 10, did a great job)
   Proactiv Solution, 4.4; benzoyl peroxide–allylamine, 6.6
8. How satisfied were you with the treatment? (1, not at all; 10, very satisfied)
   Proactiv Solution, 4.5; benzoyl peroxide–allylamine, 7.5
9. Would you like to continue the treatment after the study is over? (1, no; 10, definitely)
   Proactiv Solution, 5.4; benzoyl peroxide–allylamine, 6.6
10. How would you rate your improvement in feeling more comfortable and confident around other people as a result of treatment? (1, no change; 10, significantly improved)
    Proactiv Solution, 3.4; benzoyl peroxide–allylamine, 5.6

database Medline to support this low level of glycolic acid—therefore, it might be a good time to redirect some of that TV marketing money into product research. It is also important to note that much of the published research has used a combination of glycolic acid and agents that are actually prescription items.

Some people will see dramatic improvement when these over-the-counter topicals are used on a consistent basis. However, for those who have an unsatisfactory response, dermatologists now have an array of topical products that might be prescribed. Here are the main players.

PRESCRIPTION TOPICAL TREATMENTS

1. Topical Retinoid Creams, Gels, or Liquids—These are synthetic derivatives of vitamin A, and they help regulate the overgrowth of the cells that line the follicle. This, in turn, helps to prevent the cellular buildup and blockage that result in comedones. The topical retinoids have been a cornerstone of acne therapy for the last thirty years. The research supporting the use of the three main topical retinoids (tretinoin, adapalene, and tazarotene) is very compelling and should be expected to lead to a 50 percent improvement in cases of mild to moderate acne. For some, topical retinoids can be hard to use because for the first several weeks the skin can become red, dry, and irritated. Topical retinoids might cause a flare-up or worsening of the appearance of acne in the first four to six weeks as part of the healing process with the existing acne.

2. Topical Antibiotic Creams, Lotions, Solutions—These are agents that wipe out the bacteria associated with acne. The antimicrobial effect against P. acnes translates into a reduction in the number of lesions formed. Since many antibiotics, including topicals, have an anti-inflammatory effect, this may be an additional mechanism to explain efficacy. One of the drawbacks of topical antibiotic treatment is that the benefits decline over time—this is probably a result of the increased resistance of the bacteria P. acnes to the antibiotics. Simply put, the bacteria wise up and learn how to overcome the antimicrobial effect over time. Many new studies suggest a benefit to combining the topical antibiotic preparations with other topicals including benzoyl peroxide and retinoids. Still, application of topical antibiotics should not be a long-term thing and should be discontinued after six to eight weeks or as soon as marked improvement occurs, whichever comes first. Topical antibiotics can find their way into wide-

spread circulation throughout the body, and, although rare, cases of colitis resulting from topical use have been reported.

In cases of moderate to severe acne, your dermatologist also has prescription drug options for internal use. These agents are known as systemic because they work through the bloodstream and address acne from the inside out.

PRESCRIPTION SYSTEMIC TREATMENTS

1. Oral Antibiotics—As you might imagine, antibiotics taken by mouth can reduce the number of P. acnes that reside in the pilosebaceous units. It is quite amazing, really, that an internally consumed antibiotic can influence the bacteria that reside at the most external reaches of the body. In addition to attacking the bacteria, antibiotics also have a significant anti-inflammatory activity that may help to improve acne. Despite being used for decades, there is relatively little solid research from randomized, controlled trials (RCT) documenting the benefit of oral anti-biotics in acne. This was acknowledged recently in one of the largest reviews on acne treatments, published in the Journal of the American Medical Association (August 11, 2004). It should also be pointed out that one of the most commonly prescribed antibiotics for acne (minocycline) is completely lacking in high-quality research data when it comes to first-line therapeutic use—this from the well-known Cochrane group, which per-forms evidence-based research reviews. Here are the research-er's conclusions regarding minocycline and acne: "This review found no reliable RCT evidence to justify its continued use first-line, especially given the price differential and the concerns that still remain about its safety. Its efficacy relative to other acne therapies could not be reliably determined due to the poor methodological quality of the trials and lack of consistent choice of outcome measures."

Based on the limited data, those who use oral antibiotics should expect about a 50 percent improvement in the number of acne lesions. However, those who use long-term oral antibiotics might also expect some adverse events that should be cause for concern. For example, prior antibiotic use has been associated with increased risk of subsequent breast cancer, irritable bowel syndrome, Crohn's disease, allergies, and asthma. In addition to these research reports (referenced in the appendix), which show a general concern about the overprescribing of antibiotics, there is also evidence that extended use of antibiotics specifically prescribed for acne may cause a compromised immune system. A recent study published in the Archives of Dermatology (2005) shows that those with acne who are treated with long-term antibiotics are twice as likely to have upper respiratory tract infections when followed for one year. There is also a host of adverse reactions to antibiotics, including gastrointestinal upset, yeast overgrowths, photosensitivity, discolored teeth, and even lupus. It is becoming more and more difficult to justify the use of oral antibiotics to treat acne. As we will discuss later, the beneficial bacteria that reside in the gastrointestinal tract are wiped out with antibiotic use, and this may actually promote inflammation, increase oxidative stress, and negatively impact the healing process in acne. Some encouraging new research published in the Archives of Dermatology (2003) shows that the antibiotic doxycycline at doses 80 percent less than routinely prescribed can lead to noticeable improvements in acne lesions. At this level there is no antimicrobial effect at all, so the benefits appear to be strictly due to the anti-inflammatory mechanisms induced by the medication.

2. Hormone Therapy—Oral contraceptives (OCs) contain synthetic derivatives of the estrogens and progesterone that are made naturally in women's bodies. In many important ways they can mimic the natural molecules; however, there are also concerns. For example, OCs may cause insulin elevations and insulin resistance (which is in turn connected to unstable blood sugar, elevated blood hormone levels, and acne). Despite the adverse effect on insulin control, the acne-protective properties of OCs are dominant and appear to work through other hormonal pathways. A number of low-estrogen OCs have been shown to be helpful in females with acne. OCs work by reducing the levels of androgens that circulate through the body. Androgens are steroid hormones

(testosterone being the most well known) that stimulate the
production of sebum in both males and females. Low-estrogen
OCs increase the amount of a blood protein that binds sex hormones including testosterone, and the available evidence suggests
that this translates into about a 50 percent improvement in the
number of acne lesions. The low-estrogen OCs have a better
safety profile than standard OCs and are not associated with the
same risks of breast cancer and cardiovascular events. One of the
often overlooked consequences of binding blood testosterone in
women on even low-estrogen OCs is a markedly lowered libido.
The long-term effects of OC prescription on insulin regulation
are largely unknown, so some caution is advised when using artificial hormone manipulation as an acne treatment for years at
a time. However, it is not only estrogen that is important. The
progesterone-like part of the OCs (progestins) is also known to
be androgenic. As you know, androgen promotion fuels acne.
Recently, a non-androgenic progestin in a low-estrogren OC
called Yasmin has been approved by the FDA.

3. Isotretinoin—Isotetinoin is a vitamin A metabolite that is actually formed naturally in the human body, albeit at far lower levels
   than that used therapeutically. Marketed under the trade name
   Accutane (and its generics Amnesteem, Claravis, and Sotret),
   it is the only treatment that is considered a "cure" for acne. All
   other treatments would be considered "suppressive"—if you stop
   using them, acne will recur. More than half of the patients who
   complete a twenty-week course of Accutane (dose 0.5 to 1 mg
   per kilogram of body weight) have virtually no more acne! We
   will also learn how diet can make a difference too! For example,
   in patients who adhere to a strict, dairy-free diet, the acne recur-
   rence rate is only about 5 percent. More on that later—for now,
   back to Accutane. This is the single most effective medication
   for acne as it shrinks the sebaceous glands and addresses all the
   major processes behind the development of acne—it prevents
   overgrowth of the sebaceous gland, lowers sebum production,
   normalizes the overproduction of the cells from the follicle lining, has antioxidant and anti-inflammatory activity, and keeps *P.*

acnes growth in check. It is no wonder, then, that isotretinoin has been shown to reduce the number of acne lesions by as much as 90 percent. Despite the potential benefits, a laundry list of potential side effects, some of them very serious, has plagued the medication since its introduction in 1982. Probably the greatest concern is that related to birth defects during pregnancy—very high doses of vitamin A (and its breakdown products) are well known to be teratogenic (capable of causing fetal malformations), and the FDA has taken significant steps to prevent this from happening with young women on isotretinoin. Since major malformations occur in 40 percent of developing fetuses, strict guidelines are now in place for the use of the medication, including the iPLEDGE program with negative pregnancy tests before initiation, adequate contraception, and monthly pregnancy tests during and through six weeks after medication use. A separate area of concern relates to the case reports that suggest a link between isotretinoin and depression, suicide, panic attacks, cravings, and psychosis. The medical literature has been peppered with such reports, the first of which appeared within one year of the medication's commercial debut. A link should not be entirely surprising when one considers the published reports of vitamin A toxicity, which include depression, aggression, personality changes, cognitive difficulties, crying, feelings of guilt, and psychotic symptoms. Recently two important studies have documented potential mechanisms whereby isotretinoin might induce depressive symptoms. The first, a human study involving adults with acne, was published in the American Journal of Psychiatry (2005), and it showed that isotretinoin (vs. antibiotics) reduced metabolism in an area of the brain associated with human depression. Using sophisticated brain-imaging techniques (PET and MRI), the investigators reported a 21 percent decline in metabolic activity in a part of the frontal cortex after four months of isotretinoin. In an animal study conducted later, researchers reported in the journal Neuropsychopharmacology (2006), that six weeks of isotretinoin administration in mice produced significant changes in behavior that are consistent with human depression. The authors from the University of Texas,

Austin, point to a disruption in serotonin functioning by isotretinoin. The medication has also been reported to lower the levels
of mood-regulating vitamins B12 and folate and raise a blood
chemical called homocysteine, which has been linked with brain
disorders. Low blood levels of these two important B vitamins
have been linked to an increased risk of depression and a worse
outcome with standard treatments for depression. It appears that
isotretinoin does have biological activity within the brain, and
in certain susceptible individuals a risk of depression or other
psychological disturbances should be considered. We will discuss
the connection between the nutritional deficiencies linked to
depression and behavioral disorders, deficiencies that are strik-
ingly similar to those linked to acne. Another less appreciated
concern highlighted in the Dermatology Online Journal (2003)
is the issue of isotretinoin interfering with normal vitamin A
function. While studies have not explored this issue, case reports
suggest that isotretinoin may interfere with binding of different forms of vitamin A in the eyes and perhaps in the brain and
nerves, as well. This may help explain why we see signs of both
too much vitamin A and too little vitamin A in patients who are
taking isotretinoin. In sebaceous glands, isotretinoin binds as
vitamin A would. In the eyes, it interferes with vitamin A action
and may be evidenced as night blindness.

PHOTOTHERAPY AND HEAT TREATMENT

Specialized acne clinics are now taking advantage of light therapy in
the treatment of acne—a modern and much more refined twist on the
now abandoned ultraviolet radiation machines once used in-office by
dermatologists. Some twenty-plus light machines are now in use for
the treatment of acne, and the published research to support them
is finally starting to gain momentum. There are a few main players when it comes to light therapy machines—ultraviolet-free blue
light, red light, and intense pulsed laser. They all seem to reduce the
growth of the acne-promoting bacteria *P. acnes*. Sometimes light is
combined with topical medications for enhanced results. The benefits
might range from negligible changes to a 70 percent reduction in acne
lesions, and the side effects range from slight redness to a sunburn-like

swelling and peeling. One concern is that while they are far removed from the X-ray machines used for acne in the days of old, there have been reports of free-radical damage or excess oxidative stress in human skin exposed to the intense pulsed light. Until recently, the limited research on these so-called "optical treatments" has suffered from major design flaws. Among the newer treatments for acne, the optical treatments show significant promise. Hopefully, rigorous scientific investigations will determine the true extent of the clinical value to acne patients. Based on the evidence so far, the results of the trials and the realistic clinical value look good. It should be noted that the price tag of light therapies is high-end, anywhere from $200 to $500 per session, and is rarely covered by insurance. When it comes to acne scars, the new pulsed laser machines do offer significant hope for major improvements with resurfacing applications.

The Zeno is an exciting new handheld device about the size of a cell phone that delivers 117°C of heat to small areas of the skin for 2.5 minutes at a time. Controlled studies show that three "zaps" to a new lesion, applied at least four hours apart over twenty-four hours, are effective for many people. Application of this heat treatment works better if started soon after the lesion begins to develop. For those who have one or two lesions emerging at a time, this can be a great option. The "Zeno Effect" suggests that at least a part of the laser benefit may be derived from the local heat that lasers generate.

Washing Up

The Clear Skin Diet will devote its pages to exploring the relationship between acne, diet, and lifestyle. In particular, we will examine a lifestyle that minimizes stress and a nonrestrictive diet that promotes healthy eating habits. The message in this text will not be diluted by other far-reaching treatment techniques that may or may not be effective. There are countless over-the-counter topical preparations (scrubs, exfoliants, micropeels, goat-milk soaps, and who knows what) in department stores, supermarkets, and drugstores purported to be *the* answer to acne. Some are cheap and others are high-end, exclusive creams, gels, lotions, and potions. The really expensive ones usually come tagged with "European" or "Advanced," and the most expensive remedies are tagged as "Advanced European"—regardless of content, companies wanting to charge exorbitant amounts of money for pretty much anything in the beauty world simply list it as European.

Despite the topical-remedy overload, it is worth spending a moment on the practice of daily washing acne-prone skin. When it comes to cleansing acne-prone skin, the questions of how to wash, when to wash, how often to wash, and what to wash with have always been a matter of debate. Most of this debate has occurred outside the arena of scientific investigation; only a few studies have actually examined the practice of washing, and there really hasn't been quality research to guide patients. Dermatologists have traditionally warned against overwashing so as not to aggravate the follicles down below the pore. Harvard researchers recently examined the effect of differing washing frequency on the course of acne. Writing in the journal *Pediatric Dermatology* (2006), they reported that twice-daily washing with a mild facial cleanser (e.g., Neutrogena Fresh Foaming Cleanser) offered the greatest benefit. Specifically, Dr. Alexa Kimball and colleagues found that washing twice daily with the mild cleanser provided satisfactory results with the most improvements in open comedones and noninflammatory acne lesions. Washing only once per day was associated with a worsening of acne, while washing more than twice daily did not provide any additional benefit. Separate research published in the journal *Cutis* (2006) by Dr. Zoe Draelos showed that Cetaphil Cleanser for Normal and Oily Skin is gentle, well-tolerated, and beneficial in helping to clear up clogged pores. Many patients and dermatologists also report success with gentle cleansers from Dermalogica, a brand that includes natural botanicals, no artificial colors or fragrances (see the appendix for information on these products).

Nutritional Realities

Against the abnormal physiological processes in acne lies the context of our modern diet. It is a sad context that has been linked to many chronic diseases, most notably diabetes, cardiovascular disease, and cancer. Western nations, particularly the United States, Canada, and the United Kingdom, are not suffering from calorie deprivation. There is an abundance of food, and if we don't get a big portion size, we feel shortchanged. But what are we actually eating, and what is the nutritional quality of the supersized meals, snacks, and beverages that we hunt and gather? Simply put, there are huge nutritional voids that exist in the diets of Western nations—the research on dietary quality paints a less than flattering picture.

Consider that the most significant source of carbohydrate, cereal grains, accounts for 24 percent of our total energy intake. However, only a measly 3.5 percent of our energy from grains is accounted for by whole grains, a sad state indeed. It may seem startling that 96.5 percent of our grain intake is in the form of processed grains, especially since *whole grain* has become such a buzzword these days; however, think about the foods your local convenience store is filled with, or vending machines—foods with processed flour. When grains are processed they lose precious vitamins and minerals such as zinc, selenium, and vitamin B6, which have all been linked to protection against acne. In addition, processed grains are devoid of fiber, and in turn, missing fiber causes elevations in blood sugar and insulin release. The intake of insulin-spiking refined sugars in Western countries has increased eightfold in the last two hundred years. More recently, the intake of high-fructose corn syrup, as found in soft drinks, increased from 0.5 pound per capita in 1970 to more than 60 pounds per capita in 1997. As we will discuss later, foods that spike blood sugar and insulin release may be significant players in the production of the sebum that clogs up the follicles.

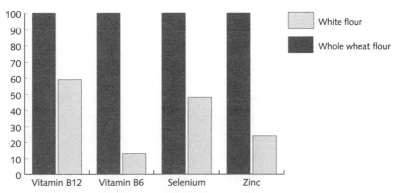

Nutrient levels after the refining of whole wheat flour. Low levels of zinc and selenium in particular have been tied to acne.

Despite the efforts of government and private nutrition education groups, and volumes of international research supporting the benefits, the fact remains that Western nations are just not eating enough fruits and vegetables. Inflated figures can be deceiving when it comes to consumption of vegetables because frozen and fried potatoes, consumed in massive amounts, are added into the data. A closer look at the vegetable data reveals shocking nutritional realities. Four foods account for half the total vegetable intake in U.S. adults—potatoes (mostly frozen and fried), iceberg lettuce, onions, and tomato. We are, of course, talking about the trimmings on a burger and a side of fries! Dark green and deep yellow vegetables, loaded with vitamin A and antioxidants, combine to account for only 6 to 8 percent of vegetable intake.

Even when potatoes and tomatoes are included, research shows that only 20 percent of adults eat the formerly recommended minimum three servings of vegetables and two servings of fruits. As of 2005, it is now recommended that we consume seven to nine servings of vegetables and fruits per day, yet 80 percent are not reaching just five servings. On a given day, almost half of all adults consume no fruit at all and, as with vegetables, variety is absent. Most fruit servings are consumed as orange juice, certainly an enjoyable and healthy beverage packed with vitamin C, but a greater variety is required to maximize health.

Children and college students also have a subpar intake of fruits and vegetables. Those in college—even when fried potatoes are included—fall short in both the fruit and vegetable categories. Of course, the students do comply with the meat (mostly high-fat, processed) and grain (mostly processed, low-fiber) group recommendations. When it comes to children, only 9 percent consume three or more servings of vegetables and two or more servings of fruits. As with adults, half of all children surveyed consumed less than one serving of fruit per day, and fried potatoes account for the majority of the vegetable intake. When fried vegetables are excluded, 30 percent of children consume less than one vegetable serving per day.

There is certainly room for improvement in the types of foods our public schools provide our teens. However, it is the so-called competitive foods that must be the starting point for reform. These are the packaged foods sold in addition to regular school lunches, in vending machines and in school shops. Their popularity has exploded in the last decade, and in many states, between 70 and 90 percent of schools have vending machines or offer separate high-fat, high-sugar snacks and beverages that compete with school lunch offerings. Research published in the *Journal of the American Dietetic Association* (2005) showed that when students choose competitive foods and beverages, they are more likely to reduce school lunch servings and take in 32 percent less of the important antioxidant and antiacne vitamin A per day. Consuming competitive foods translated into twice the sugar intake compared to those eating only the school lunches.

Nutritional doctors must face an uphill battle in educating patients in the midst of unhealthy choices. There is a massive juggernaut called the food industry, which spends $11 billion dollars annually on advertising and another $22 billion on consumer promotions. Trust us when we tell you that the fruit, vegetable, and fish portions of this massive budget amount to relative pennies. In fact, for every dollar the government spends on nutrition education, the food industry lays out twenty-four of its own dollars on marketing efforts that are rarely in sync with risk-reducing nutritional advice. Not only do subpar dietary choices surround us everywhere at all times of the day and night, the sad reality is that they are much cheaper than healthy choices. As highlighted by Dr. Sharon Wyatt and colleagues in the *American Journal of Medical Science* (2006), a person can purchase 1,500 calories for a mere $5 in a fast-food restaurant, or for even less in a grocery store. They also noted that on a per-unit-of-food-energy basis, the cost of potato chips is about 80 percent less than the cost of raw carrots! As reported in *Time* magazine (June 4, 2007), the cost of fruits and vegetables is up by 40 percent since 1985, while various meats, vegetable oils, and soft drinks have fallen between 5 and 25 percent in the same period. Consider also that some 30 percent of pediatric teaching hospitals have a branded (e.g., McDonald's) fast-food restaurant within the hospital itself. This only serves to encourage fast-food consumption and soften its image, with the perception that "hey, if this kind of food is endorsed by a hospital, it must not be so bad." We know this because Dr. Hannah Sahud and colleagues reported in *Pediatrics* (2006) that visitors to a hospital with a McDonald's inside its walls were four times more likely to consume McDonald's fast-food during a given day than visitors to a hospital without a fast-food franchise! While Dr. Sahud did not examine the specific choices of fast-food consumers in the hospital, there is an abundance of research showing that fast-food consumption is associated with greater overall calories and fat; more simple carbohydrates; and less fiber, fruits, and vegetables (with the exception of fried white potatoes).

Various websites and blogs tout organic foods, particularly fruits and vegetables, as *the* foods of choice for acne. While making efforts to choose only organic foods is worthwhile for our greater good, it is not always practical, nor is it always necessary. It is true that some, but not all, studies show that organics have higher nutrient content. However, research in the *Journal of Agricultural and Food Chemistry* (2004) showed that even though the tested organic produce had slightly higher levels of nutrients, when it came to human consumption there were no practical differences at all in the blood levels of the highlighted nutrients—vitamin C and lycopene. Both of these are antiacne nutrients that we will discuss along the way. The evidence for fruits and vegetables—organic or not—being health promoters is very solid—organic or not. Since there is no scientific evidence whatsoever that organic foods improve acne, and since the overall intake of fruits and vegetables in North America is woefully inadequate, some common sense should prevail. Not all fruits and vegetables are laden with pesticides, and since organic foods can be quite expensive, it makes sense to prioritize and perhaps choose to buy organic for only those fruits and vegetables with the highest levels of pesticides/herbicides. While this may not help with acne, it may influence other aspects of health, including the long-term risk of neurodegenerative diseases. In considering which fruits and vegetables to prioritize, be guided by the lists here and any updated information provided by the experts at the Environmental Working Group (www.ewg.org).

Consider that large population surveys, including the National Health and Nutrition Examination Survey and others, show at least half of the U.S. population does not meet the recommended dietary allowance (RDA) for important vitamins and minerals, including calcium, magnesium, zinc, vitamin A, and vitamin B6. These are the minimal recommended intakes! Low dietary zinc in particular is

Most Contaminated Foods	Least Contaminated Foods
apples	asparagus
bell peppers	avocado
celery	banana
cherries	broccoli
grapes (imported)	cauliflower
nectarines	corn
peaches	kiwi
pears	mango
potatoes	onions
red raspberries	papaya
spinach	pineapple
strawberries	peas

worrisome because research shows that it is helpful in the treatment of acne. Recent studies have shown that low levels of zinc are also associated with fatigue, depression, and poor mental performance. Yet in our society we tend to bypass the dietary solution of whole grains, nuts, and seafood, and instead reach for a sugar-laden commercial energy drink.

Avoidance of a variety of fruits and vegetables and whole grains also translates into less protective dietary antioxidants. Plant foods are known to contain not only vitamins and minerals, but also more than twenty-five thousand microchemicals that give plants their color, taste, and texture. These naturally occurring chemicals are called phytochemicals, and include colorful plant pigments that have potent antioxidant activities. Phytochemicals are manufactured in plants as a defense mechanism for the purpose of their own survival and health. Most of the research on phytochemicals shows them to be protective against cardiovascular disease and various cancers; however, research also suggests great potential against acne as well.

One of the largest and best-known groups of phytochemicals is the polyphenol group. Within this family are the flavonoids, which include flavones, flavonols, flavanones, catechins, anthocyanins, and isoflavones. To provide a full spectrum of phytochemical protection, we need to consume a variety of fruits, vegetables, and plant-based beverages. For example, the catechins are found in high amounts in green tea; the anthocyanins in blueberries, cherries, and elderberries; the isoflavones in soy; the flavonols in apples; and so on. There are other important groups of phytochemicals, including the carotenoid family, which is made up of beta-carotene, lutein, lycopene, and zeaxanthin. Beta-carotene is found in carrots and other orange vegetables, lutein in dark greens such as broccoli and kale, lycopene in red vegetables such as red peppers and tomatoes, and zeaxanthin in yellow vegetables and greens such as corn and spinach. In addition, there are other beneficial phytochemicals such as limonene in citrus fruits, ellagic acid in berries, and sulforaphane in Brussels sprouts, kale, cabbage, and broccoli. Antioxidants work together in a synergistic fashion, and without a broad range of colorful foods, we are not taking full advantage of nature's protective chemicals.

There has also been a marked decrease in the intake of omega-3 essential fatty acids over the last hundred years. These essential fats have important anti-inflammatory activities that hold great promise in the treatment of acne. At the same time there has been a significant increase in the supply of vegetable oils such as corn, safflower, sunflower, and soybean oils which supply omega-6 linoleic acid. Too much linoleic acid and too little omega-3 are well documented to promote inflammation. The North American omega-6 intake is now outnumbering omega-3 intake by a ratio as high as 20:1. This current ratio is quite a distance from the ideal ratio of 2:1 (omega-6 to omega-3) recommended by an international panel of lipid experts in the

Top Food Choices as Reported by 227 Public High School Food-Service Directors (Adapted from Probart et al., *J Am Diet Assoc* 2005)

1. Pizza, hamburgers, and sandwiches
2. Cookies, crackers, and fat-containing baked goods
3. Fried potatoes
4. Salty, fat-containing snacks
5. Sweetened beverages

Journal of the American College of Nutrition (1999). The average daily intake of combined EPA/DHA in the United States is only 130 mg, which is more than 500 mg short of published recommendations and close to 900 mg short of the 1000 mg recommended by the American Heart Association in cases of heart disease. A recent Canadian study showed that pregnant women consume an average of 80 mg of DHA per day, well short of the minimum 300 mg recommended for fetal and early childhood development.

In addition to the nutritional voids of vitamins, minerals, omega-3 fatty acids, and phytochemicals, a fourth gaping hole is that of fiber intake. Fiber is the component of plants that the human body is unable to digest—it is also the component of grains that is lost in processing. Dietary fiber intake is subpar, and its absence, as we will discuss, may have acne implications way beyond the gastrointestinal tract. North Americans are consuming only 13 grams of fiber per day—at least 33 percent less than traditional diets consumed a century ago. We should be anywhere from 7 to 25 g higher, depending on age and gender.

Depending on an individual's genetic makeup, nutritional voids and dietary excesses may influence whether or not an individual experiences acne, or the degree to which one experiences acne. There are some people on this earth who will never experience acne, you know, the friend we all know from high school who ate whatever he liked—chips, processed foods, fatty foods, chocolate, sweets, and soft drinks—without even so much as a whitehead. These people are like the proverbial heavy smokers who live a full life to the age of ninety and die peacefully in their sleep. Not every person will experience acne with unhealthy eating habits, although, if you are reading this book, you are not likely one of them. The vast majority of unhealthy eaters will succumb to nutritional influences on genetics (i.e., the influences of saturated fats and sugars—and the absence of protective vitamins, minerals, good fats, fiber, and phytochemicals—on the genetic expression of chemicals and enzymes that control the risk and physiological processes of cardiovascular disease, cancer, diabetes, and . . . acne).

Thanks to emerging research in the discipline known as "nutritional genomics" (or nutrigenomics), we now know that nutrition plays a role in whether or not, and to what degree, an illness may present itself. Consider diabetes (type 2), where healthy dietary modifications can reverse the illness in some individuals. In this case, the expression of genetic information is altered by changing one environmental variable. In diabetes, and very likely in acne also, the one environmental variable that can influence the disease onset, and/or its course, is nutrition.

Consider that 99.9 percent of all humans are identical in terms of gene sequence, however, the 0.1 percent variation in sequence accounts for differences in our appearance and, notably, our susceptibility to disease. Acne is, undoubtedly, strongly influenced by genetics. However, if genetics were the whole story, then identical twins (who share exactly the same gene sequence) would always have the same degree of acne as they proceed through life—they don't. As highlighted in a recent study in the *British Journal of Dermatology* (2005), the genetic influence on acne varies with age, gender, and location of the acne lesions so that the genetic influence might lie somewhere between 31 and 97 percent. That is a pretty broad range, and one that leaves quite a bit of room for environmental influences, including nutrition, stress, and lifestyle. All too often conditions like acne are written off as genetic, implying that there is nothing one can do to alter them. However, we are now learning that genes can indeed be influenced by diet and lifestyle. This emerging and exciting area of nutritional science is termed *nutrigenomics*.

Caveat

We need to emphasize one caveat that relates to the unknowns of acne. At this point researchers do not understand all the factors and processes that combine to cause acne. A greater knowledge of the human genome has given us some pieces of the puzzle. We know, for example, that some people have difficulty with the processing of vitamin A, while others metabolize hormones too slowly. Some of these unique physiological influences will respond to nutritional interventions such as increasing vitamin A. It is anticipated that a single drop of blood will provide answers for sophisticated interventions based on the genetic profile. Yet this may be decades away, and, for now, we must recognize that while most people will see improvement with the diet and lifestyle changes we propose, a few will not. They may find that their overall health, energy levels, and perhaps mental outlook improve, yet the acne stubbornly persists. These patients need the "big guns" in the dermatological arsenal and should not hesitate to seek appropriate dermatological care. Everyone, whether they have acne or not, can benefit from the healthy eating and lifestyle habits presented later in the Clear Skin Diet Action Plan.

Chapter Key Points

✓ Acne incidence is on the rise globally.

✓ Increased rates of acne are not due to genetic changes; all arrows point to changes in our lifestyle or environment.

✓ Diet and nutrition, although refuted and rejected without adequate testing, may be a major player in acne for most people.

✓ Acne is characterized by increased sebum (oil) production from the sebaceous glands in the skin, occlusion or clogging of the follicle (pore), and within the ducts, an overgrowth of bacteria that normally reside on the skin.

✓ The process promotes inflammation and oxidative (free-radical) stress.

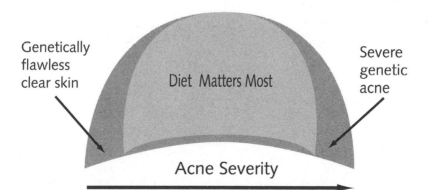

The Curve of Acne—At one end are the lucky ones who laugh in the face of fast food, fats, and sugar—they seem totally immune to acne. At the other are those afflicted with the most severe forms of acne, and, despite making the best efforts, diet just doesn't seem to play a large role in some cases.

✓ Comedones can present in the open form (blackheads) or the closed form (whiteheads).

✓ Papules are elevated red bumps and pustules including a collection of white blood cells and bacteria that present as yellowish pus.

✓ Nodules are large, painful, deeply formed bumps that may leave a scar with improper healing.

✓ Standard treatments include over-the-counter topicals—benzoyl peroxide, salicylic acid, glycolic acid—and prescription topicals—retinoic acids or antibiotics. Oral prescriptions include anti-biotics, hormones, and isotretinoin. Phototherapy—light treatment—is an emerging therapy.

✓ Gentle cleansing twice per day is valuable.

✓ Many people skip nutritious foods that would otherwise fulfill the minimum recommended dietary allowances.

✓ Western nations are overconsuming vegetable oils and sidestepping healthy omega-3 fatty acids.

✓ The typical Western diet is lacking in fiber and deeply colored fruits and vegetables.

2

Nutritional Medicine and Acne

THE AREA OF RESEARCH AND clinical work governing nutritional influences on health has rapidly grown into its own discipline called nutritional medicine. There are now volumes of international research that document the powerful influence of dietary choices on human health. To one degree or another, dietary quality (or the lack thereof) can influence most chronic diseases—both in risk of onset and the general outcome of a condition. The connections between nutrition and health are perhaps most well recognized in the areas of cardio-vascular disease, diabetes, obesity, cancer, and brain degenerative diseases later in life. The connection between nutrition and psychiatric conditions, particularly depression and childhood behavioral disorders, has picked up considerable steam in recent years. Sophisticated scientific investigations have now documented mechanisms behind the nutritional influences on the main players in most chronic conditions—genetics, oxidative stress, and inflammation. The advances in nutritional medicine have wide-ranging applications in human health, including the health of the human skin. Sadly, many in the modern dermatology profession remain resistant to nutritional advances, particularly when it comes to acne.

A study published in the *Australasian Journal of Dermatology* (2001) showed that almost half of fourth-year medical students (on the eve of graduation) considered diet to be an important factor in acne. The researchers, from the Department of Dermatology of the University of Melbourne, considered such a high percentage of new doctors (non-dermatologists) linking diet and acne as "cause for concern." They went on to say that the diet-acne link was a result of the misconceptions of the general community, which "strongly implanted the idea among medical students who were unsuccessfully disabused during their training." It's pretty hard to disabuse someone about diet and acne when the actual misconception is that there is solid evidence showing an absence of a relationship between diet and acne. Despite all that is known in the area of nutritional medicine today, why on earth does the dermatological community continue to relegate dietary influences on acne to "myth" status? How is it that no matter where the study is conducted—United States, Canada, Australia, United Kingdom, New Zealand, Sweden, Nigeria, Germany, Japan, Jordan, or Saudi Arabia (in other words, pretty much all parts of the globe)—the majority of those with acne suspect diet to be involved as a causative or therapeutic factor? Is it because acne patients are delusional? In the 1970s the prevailing attitude was just that, with one dermatologist stating in the journal *American Family Physician* in 1971, "Too many patients harbor the delusion that their health can somehow be mysteriously harmed by something in their diet." Then we have renowned dermatologist Albert Kligman, quoted in *the* acne textbook for dermatologists of the 1970s (*Acne: Morphogenesis and Treatment*, Springer-Verlag 1975), who suggested that dietary restrictions or removal of what he called "tempting delights" to deal with teen acne, were a purposeful means to punish sexually driven teens. He contended that the removal of pleasurable foods (presumably high-fat and high-sugar foods) were measures fabricated by parents and doctors "to keep these imminent sinners in check." We couldn't disagree more, although, in fairness, we have the advantage of observing massive advances in the field of nutrition since the 1970s.

In his acne textbook, Dr. Kligman went on to acknowledge that some patients did get worse after consuming so-called tempting delights, and this, he said, was due to anxious and tense patients who subsequently picked and squeezed at their skin—making tiny acne lesions into large ones. So dermatologists were being taught two things at this time—first and foremost, that there is no connection between diet and acne; and second, that any flare-up after consuming high-fat, high-sugar foods is entirely a result of the patient's beliefs and anxious behavior. In Dr. Logan's own experiences with acne, he never picked or squeezed lesions, big or small, so he can say with confidence that he was not picking his way to acne flare-ups after eating less-than-healthy foods.

Why is it that dermatology dogma tells us we all are individually and collectively wrong? Why is it that some dermatologists are in vehement opposition to the very suggestion that diet and acne might be related? There are a number of factors involved, including lack of nutritional training in medical schools and dermatology residency programs, two poorly designed and implemented studies that were interpreted as demonstrating no connection between diet and acne, and, of course, some of the more vocal acne-drug advocates have to protect their interest in patented formulations from the threat of a non-pharmacologic therapy. As time went by, the beliefs and opinions of the dermatologists grew stronger and they became a collective professional reality—and let's face it, after almost forty years of taking a strong stance against any possible relationship between diet and acne, it is hard to say, "Wait a minute—we may have to re-think this."

Lack of Nutritional Training

The first block to nutritional counseling in acne is, as mentioned, related to inadequate training of our doctors. There are exceptions to the rule; there is a small minority of MDs who practice holistic dermatology, and these specialists have trained in nutritional medicine staying current with the latest advances. These few dermatologists have understood that the onus has been on them to pursue an education in nutritional medicine. Why? Holistic dermatologists openly admit, and the research shows, nutritional training certainly wasn't provided during the years of medical school and dermatology residency. How can dermatologists be expected to provide counsel on nutrition in general, let alone in acne, if they are never taught even basic clinical nutrition? Conventional medicine can work near miracles, and dermatology has its well-researched share of extraordinary treatments. However, for the more chronic conditions such as acne, a more holistic approach may add great value to overall care. Incorporating nutrition, mind-body medicine, counseling, stress management, acupuncture, and other such approaches along with the best that modern, mainstream dermatology has to offer expands the medicinal toolbox.

A variety of research studies show that medical students and residents within specialties barely even touch on nutrition. The largest survey to date, published in *Medical Education Online* (1998), showed that only 55 percent of medical schools in the United States had an actual nutrition course. Only 7 percent of the schools had a *clinical practice* nutrition course to give future MDs the chance to get into nutrition from a clinical or hands-on perspective. Regarding the total hours of nutrition education, 75 percent of the schools required courses that amounted to only twenty or fewer hours. The few hours spent on nutrition in most medical schools is related to biochemical reactions of the energy cycle in the human cells (the Krebs cycle) and the use of lifesaving IV nutrition within hospital settings—so it's not the *clinical* nutrition education related to chronic diseases that would serve to benefit the patients in day-to-day practice. A more recent survey in the *American Journal of Clinical Nutrition* (2006) indicates that not much has changed since 1998—nutritional training remains woefully inadequate, and only 30 percent of medical schools require an actual nutrition course. In the same issue of the journal, it was reported that 78 percent of graduating medical students do not believe they were extensively trained in nutritional counseling, and only 17 percent frequently counseled their patients on nutrition. In their own daily living, only 11 percent of the students met the U.S. national guideline of even the minimal intake of five servings of fruits and vegetables per day. Interestingly, the med students who were going on to specialize in an area of medicine (that would include dermatology) were the least interested in nutritional counseling. It appears that some students heading for dermatology and other specialty areas had already made up their minds to shut the door on the relevance of nutrition in medicine.

This is a pretty sad state of affairs, fed by virtually no accountability for nutritional knowledge via licensing exams. Research shows that only 3 percent of six thousand medical licensing board exam questions are even remotely related to nutrition. Why bother learning about it if you aren't going to be tested on it? All of this sets a tone about nutrition—if it is not prioritized in the four years of basic medical education and advanced specialty training, if it is glossed over, if competency is not examined, then how important can nutrition really be? It also translates into a lack of knowledge about nutrition.

Two separate studies in the *Nutrition Journal* (2003 and 2005) investigated the basic nutritional knowledge of medical students and internists and found huge gaping holes in even the fundamentals of nutrition. From correctly identifying good sources of monounsaturated fats, to the influences of fats and carbohydrates on cholesterol and triglyceride levels, the results were, let's just say, alarming. More than one-quarter of the med students did not know that fat contains, gram-for-gram, more calories than an equivalent serving of carbohydrates or protein. Three-quarters were unaware that canola oil is a good source of monounsaturated fat, and about half the students were unaware that olive oil is rich in monounsaturated fat. Almost half of the med students thought that folic acid supplementation can make up for a vitamin B12 deficiency, and 75 percent were unaware that vitamin B12 deficiency is commonly observed in the elderly due to poor absorption. We are willing to cut the med students some slack because they are, after all, students—but clearly they need some serious "disabuse."

In the study involving the seasoned physicians specializing in internal medicine, half were unable to correctly identify the oils that are good sources of monounsaturated fat. Ninety-three percent (84 percent of cardiologists vs. 96 percent of internists) did not know the effects of a low-fat diet on blood triglycerides. Approximately three-quarters (70 percent of cardiologists vs. 77 percent of internists) did not know the effects of a low-fat diet on HDL (the "good") cholesterol. With this unimpressive background in mind, you may want to think twice if you are dismissed with the "no relationship between acne and diet" line as if it were indeed fact.

In the interest of being complete, we will point out that both authors of *The Clear Skin Diet* have taken advanced clinical nutrition training. Dr. Treloar has countless hours of approved continuing medical education credits in nutrition and is among the few medical doctors with the Certified Nutrition Specialist status granted through the American College of Nutrition. As for Dr. Logan, nutrition is the foundation stone of his field of naturopathic medicine—transcripts from his four years of naturopathic medical school show 223 required hours of classroom nutritional education, not including hundreds of hours in clinical practicum. In addition, licensure as a naturopathic physician in the select states and provinces where there are laws governing practice requires the passage of individual board exams where 100 percent of the exam questions are specifically on biochemical and *clinical* nutrition.

Naturopathic medicine is a discipline that supports the healing process in a holistic fashion, one that considers lifestyle, stressors, and nutrition to be of major importance. In addition to the nutritional training, naturopathic physicians do have the luxury of time—they spend about forty-five minutes with each patient. According to a University of Toronto study published in the journal *Pediatrics* (2005), 23 percent of all childhood and teen visits to a large naturopathic clinic are for the treatment of skin conditions. It is likely that many parents seek to take advantage of the nutritional interventions that often make up the treatment protocol for skin conditions, including acne. Research also shows that among patients with skin conditions, those with acne have the greatest confidence in complementary approaches.

It is, however, important to underscore that alternatives are not a substitute for medical/dermatological evaluation and care. Nutrition and other adjuvant approaches work most efficiently for skin care when combined with the conventional approaches of your dermatologist. Diet and lifestyle change may allow you and your doctor to decrease your doses or frequency of medical treatment. They may also allow for medications to be discontinued more rapidly, although this should always be discussed with your provider. Despite the shortcomings in nutritional training, remember that no other health-care provider has the extensive training in the recognition of skin lesions that your dermatologist has. You really want to be sure that you do not have an "acne mimic," a different condition that might respond to separate treatment or one that might be an indicator of a systemic disease. Modern dermatology is a profession in the business of saving and improving lives; therefore, when any skin condition develops it should be evaluated first by the experts.

Patent Protection

Now, back to the reasons why the diet-acne connection has been relegated to a nonissue in dermatology. Over the past few decades, the pharmaceutical industry has become an ever more important source of funding for medical research, postgraduate training, and continuing medical education. As with medicine in general, dermatology has been influenced by the dramatic and profitable growth of the pharmaceutical industry. The end result is the development of pharmaco-dermatologists who wield powerful prescription pads. Consider that in the February 2007 issue of the *Archives of Dermatology* there are seventy-four pages of glossy pharmaceutical advertisements and eighty-five pages of scientific papers. Throw in an additional twelve pages of nondrug ads, and the end result is that marketing tips the scale compared to the scientific papers. We should also point out that of the studies investigating drugs or devices, financial sponsorship of the study or scientist is commonplace.

Thankfully, researchers such as Dr. Loren Cordain from Colorado State University and others from Harvard Medical School have taken up the torch to investigate a diet-acne connection. They found one, and it shook up many in the dermatology community. Some reacted to evidence connecting diet and acne as if it were a personal assault to the dermatology community and its long-term stance against such a connection. It was also a threat to the pharmaceutical industry because the studies confirmed what people in the non-dermatologic community have known for years—diet matters. Some made various futile attempts to discredit the recent diet-acne research, most displaying a clear lack of knowledge when it comes to the influences of nutrition on physiology and human genetics.

To witness the influence of diet on human genetics, one need only look to Japan, home of the largest nutritional experiment ever conducted. In just a few short decades, the Japanese have grown taller, stronger, and wider (young women are the exception due to social pressure to remain thin). There have been remarkable changes to the Japanese diet, with significant increases in the dietary intake of milk, meat, animal fat, processed foods, and sugar. The cholesterol levels of young Japanese are now barely indistinguishable from North Americans'—they were once miles apart. We have known for quite some time that when residents of Japan move to North America they experience increased rates of genetically influenced conditions including cardiovascular disease and Parkinson's disease. The downside to the rapid dietary changes inside Japan are the major increases in chronic disease states within the nation—and, yes, there has also been an increase in the prevalence of acne, which we will discuss in detail later.

The Two Old Studies

Among those who suspect that dietary factors are involved in the exacerbation and improvement of acne, many report chocolate as a culprit. With this in mind, two studies were conducted to determine if chocolate bars might influence the development or aggravation of acne. The first, in 1969 by Fulton, Plewig, and Kligman, looked at the daily consumption of a 112 g bar of bittersweet chocolate for one month. There were sixty-five teens and adults enrolled in the trial, and those not eating the bittersweet were given an identical-looking "placebo" bar that did not contain the chocolate liquor (aka cacao paste) that is typical of a commercial chocolate bar. The authors of the study concluded that the ingestion of chocolate did not influence the course of acne over a month relative to the placebo.

But did they really investigate the influence of chocolate on acne? More than 50 percent of chocolate liquor consists of lipids (fats), the vast majority of which are saturated fats. Since saturated fats were getting the negative press in the late 1960s and early 1970s, and hydrogenated oils were all the rage, it made sense at the time to make the placebo bar with "healthy" vegetable oil and not the saturated fats found in chocolate. Through the wonders of modern food processing, we can make vegetable oils solid at room temperature by hydrogenation. However, when vegetable oils are hydrogenated there is also the formation of undesirable trans fats, so Fulton's placebo bar was far from healthy—we now know these trans fats are even worse than saturated fats when it comes to human health. Here is what the prestigious Institute of Medicine has to say about them: "Saturated fats, trans fatty acids, and dietary cholesterol have no known beneficial role in preventing chronic disease and are not required at any level in the diet. . . . The recommendation is to keep their intake as low as possible." (*Institute of Medicine* 2002, Dietary Reference Intakes for Energy, Carbohydrate, Fiber, Fatty Acids, Cholesterol, Protein, Amino Acids). Research indicates that our bodies really don't know what to make of trans fats, and they really wreak havoc, promoting inflammation, elevating cholesterol, and increasing the risk of diabetes. Gram-for-gram, trans fats increase the risk of cardiovascular blockage by more than tenfold versus saturated fats. So Fulton and his colleagues created a placebo look-alike bar that was arguably even worse than the chocolate bar itself. As far as the total fat and sugar content of the two bars, there really was no difference at all between the two.

It might be unfair for us to hold the researchers to the high standard of nutritional knowledge that has since emerged some thirty-plus years after their work. However, just five years after the chocolate study, Dr. Bruce Mackie, who was the chairman of dermatology at the Prince of Wales Hospital in Sydney, Australia, and dietician Leila Mackie examined the issue of the makeup of the placebo bar. They wrote a scathing critical review of the Fulton study and highlighted the fact that it basically compared apples to apples. Writing in the *Australasia Journal of Dermatology* (1974), they stated, "If the work of Fulton is now examined in light of these facts it becomes apparent that their trial feeding of chocolate was incorrectly controlled and their results are therefore not valid." Sadly, no one was listening and the damage had been done; dermatologists looked at the Fulton study and took the lack of connection between chocolate and acne as fact. The Fulton study was then extrapolated to mean that there is no connection between *any* foods and acne.

There were other critics as well, including Dr. James Rasmussen, a dermatologist from the University of Michigan. It was he who criticized the study design itself, in particular that the Fulton study relied upon comedones (black and whiteheads) as an outcome measure, which diluted the data on so-called pustular flares. Rather than blackheads, the larger red acne lesions with visible pus (hence the name pustular flares) are more characteristic of reactions to certain foods. Since he was counting blackheads and whiteheads and throwing them together into the total before-and-after outcome pot, Fulton's methods were probably not sensitive enough to pick up the changes in the more visible pustular flares. If he and his colleagues had looked at exclusively pustular flares we would actually put our money down on the hydrogenated/trans-fat placebo bar being even worse than the real chocolate bar at promoting acne! Further, it should be noted that this was only a six-week study in which the endpoint was comedo formation, something that can take months to truly develop. The time allowed was far too short for the outcome chosen.

Two years after the Fulton study came another chocolate and acne study by Philip Anderson. When you don't blind a study and you are the sole investigator, as in this case, research shows that even unintentional investigator bias creeps in like a poison. Anderson was an outspoken critic of any chocolate-acne connection—he had stated six years earlier in the *Missouri Medicine* journal (1965) that there was no connection, so he entered the study with a documented bias. Anderson gathered twenty-seven medical students who reported worsening of acne after the ingestion of either chocolate, milk, cola, or peanuts. Before he challenged the students with the offending foods, he put a see-through plastic sheet over each subject's face and marked the acne lesions with a pencil. Over the course of the week the students were asked to consume liberal amounts of the offending foods—depending on the reported offender, this involved supervised daily doses of six small chocolate bars, a quart of milk, four ounces of peanuts, or two cans of cola. The milk and cola groups were asked to consume an additional quart of milk or two cans of cola on their own. Anderson reported that the dietary challenges made no overall difference after the week or ten days. We have no idea how many people were in each group, and since there were only twenty-seven students to begin with, it is unlikely that any group had enough statistical power to provide meaningful results. In other words, if only four students were in the cola group, this would not be enough to tell us anything more than what might happen by chance alone after cola drinking. Anderson did not report on changes to any particular lesion type (pustular flares, for example) and did not subject his results to statistical analysis. Then there is the issue of control groups (i.e., comparative subjects with either a separate or no acne intervention). Oops, there was no control group with which to compare the students! With the small size, lack of a control group, and open design, this paper would probably not be accepted for publication today. However, perhaps the biggest gaping hole in this study was that the students' backgrounds or baseline diets were not evaluated. In all probability, their diets were a high-carbohydrate "dorm diet," the implications of which we will discuss later when we touch on blood sugar and acne. Fulton's chocolate-and-acne study had the same major oversight of not knowing what else the participants were eating and drinking during the course of the study. Again, the time frame to observe changes was inappropriate; even giving an extra quart of milk for one week would have had minimal effect in this brief study.

Despite the design flaws that basically render the conclusions null and void, these two studies continue to be used as the proof that there is no relationship between chocolate and the onset or course of acne. Chocolate may or may not *aggravate* acne—it probably depends on the individual—however, an even greater concern is that these studies are also used as evidence that there is no relationship between overall dietary quality and acne. Obviously, if these two studies cannot tell us anything about the relationship between chocolate and acne, they should never be used to claim that diet itself has no bearing on acne.

Chocolate actually comes in many different forms, with vastly different ingredient profiles: milk chocolate, white chocolate, a chocolate coating (as well as chocolate flavored chips, shavings, and bits) rich in hydrogenated, inflammation-promoting trans fats. These may be the forms of chocolate those with acne refer to as offending foods. On the other hand, dark chocolate (with at least 70 percent cocoa) and pure cocoa powder may not be involved, or, better yet, they may even be influencing acne for the better! Wait, we know what you're thinking—how could we make such a statement after critically dismantling the two chocolate-acne studies?

The nutritional profile of dark chocolate, with a 70 percent minimum cocoa content and cocoa itself, is very different from milk chocolate, radically different from white chocolate, and light-years away from those trans fat–laden chocolate coatings/bits. Cocoa, and dark chocolate rich in cocoa, contains naturally occurring antioxidant and anti-inflammatory chemicals called flavonoids. When foods are coated with milk and white chocolate, or when the bits are added, not only are there little to no flavonoids, there are also the inflammation and oxidative stress promoting trans/saturated fats and sugar. We will discuss how foods that promote inflammation and oxidative stress have the potential to adversely affect acne.

A growing number of human studies have shown that dark chocolate rich in flavonoids or high-flavonoid cocoa drinks can improve blood flow to skin cells, prevent oxidative stress to fatty components of cells, improve hydration and texture of skin, and prevent skin damage associated with ultraviolet rays. A recent study in the *American Journal of Clinical Nutrition* (2005) showed that dark chocolate improves how our bodies respond to the blood-sugar-regulating hormone insulin, and, as we will see, this would benefit acne. In addition, two groundbreaking studies, one in the *European Journal of Nutrition* (2006) and the other in the *Journal of Nutrition* (2006), show that cocoa powder rich in flavonoids can improve blood flow to the skin and improve skin hydration in adult women. Since we are now close to being forty years removed from these chocolate-acne studies, it might be time to repeat them with scientific rigor, and it may be worthwhile to compare a high-flavonoid dark chocolate bar or cocoa-powder drink with one containing only the milk, sugar, and saturated fats. At this point it would be unethical to design a placebo bar with trans/hydrogenated fats since we know with great certainty how damaging they can be.

The Irony of Iodine

Despite the distancing between the profession and any diet-acne connection whatsoever, one nutrient continues to be vilified as a causative factor in acne. Despite very compelling and solid research to the contrary, even some of North America's most famous dermatologists warn that iodine from fish, seafood, and seaweed causes acne. So we have a situation where those with acne are told that diet doesn't matter, but hey, watch out for fish and seafood because iodine causes acne. The reality, as pointed out by Dr. F. William Danby in the *Journal of the American Academy of Dermatology* (2007), is that there is no evidence to support iodides as the cause of acne. If an individual eats excessive amounts of iodine-rich foods (let's say, bags of the seaweed kelp), they will likely experience an acneiform eruption (i.e., something that looks a bit like acne). However, this is not acne, and there would be absolutely no signs of the classic comedones that are the hallmark of acne.

Drs. Joseph Hitch and Bernard Greenburg from the University of North Carolina conducted the largest study to determine if there is some sort of fish/seafood-iodine connection. They looked at the rates of acne in more than one thousand teenagers residing in three different locales of North Carolina—coastal dwellers, inland dwellers and those living in the mountains. To level the playing field, they made sure there were equal numbers of country (rural) and city kids in each regional group so they were not comparing rural vs. urban, and they also matched the socioeconomic backgrounds of the teens within the regions. Of course, as you might imagine, the coastal dwellers were big consumers of saltwater fish, seafood, and iodine. Amazingly, though, it was the coastal dwellers in the "high"-iodine diet who actually had the lowest prevalence of oily skin, comedones, papules, pustules, and acne cysts. Every sign of acne, with the exception of acne scars, was significantly lower among the teens eating the high-iodine saltwater fish diet and drinking the higher-iodine local water. These results, along with others, certainly negate an acne-iodine connection, yet they also hold the key to a nutritional component in acne prevention—omega-3 fatty acids. The teens consuming the diet with lots of saltwater fish and seafood were undoubtedly consuming a diet with much higher levels of critically important omega-3 fatty acids. When the study was published in the *Archives of Dermatology* (1961), scientists knew virtually nothing about these important fatty acids, so the study was basically a call to move on from this iodine-acne thinking and it was pretty much left at that. Today, with the wealth of research and awareness of omega-3 fatty acids, this large study would be seen in a different light. The connection between a diet high in saltwater fish/seafood, the obvious omega-3 content of such a diet, and a low presentation of acne would be readily apparent to researchers. As we will discuss in the next chapter, omega-3 fatty acids emerge strongly as a candidate component in the acne-protective clear skin diet.

The Three New Studies

An opinion and commentary piece appeared in the *Archives of Dermatology* (1981) under the heading "Acne Diet Reconsidered." It was written by noted dermatologist E. William Rosenberg, of the University of Tennessee, and his colleague Betsy S. Kirk, and together they made an excellent point in following the cardinal rule of epidemiology (population) studies. They underscored that the primary factor in a disease is the one where in its absence the disease will not occur. Put simply by the authors, "We could make a good case for diet as primary for acne if we could demonstrate enough absence of the disease in populations whose diets are unlike those of people in the West." This is exactly what Dr. Loren Cordain and his international team of physicians and scientists did when they put the acne-diet connection back on the scientific map. In 2002 they broke the eerie silence of research since the old chocolate studies, and they answered Dr. E. William Rosenberg's call for epidemiological examination in a publication that would be a turning point in a new era of dermatology.

We applaud the 2002 editors of the *Archives of Dermatology* who gave this controversial study the green light for publication, a particularly bold move when considering the research team did not include a dermatologist. Primary-care physicians among the team examined the prevalence of acne in two different communities that still remain relatively untouched by Western dietary influences. Specifically, they looked at the Kitavan Islanders of Papua New Guinea, and the Aché community of Paraguay; and although these groups are geographically separated by ten thousand miles, the common link is the almost exclusive consumption of nonprocessed, locally caught or cultivated foods. The Kitavans, a group with extremely low rates of chronic diseases and abdominal obesity, consume a diet primarily consisting of fish, roots, fruits, and coconuts. The Aché, a people who also have low rates of chronic diseases, consume a diet rich in wild game, small-scale local farmed goods, nuts, and foraged roots. The overall influence of processed foods, dairy, added oils, margarines, and sugars was reported to be near nil in the Kitavan diet, and around 8 percent among the Aché.

After careful dermatological examination of 300 Kitavans ages fifteen to twenty-five, there wasn't a single case of acne, not even a pustular flare to be seen! The same observation was made among the Aché; in this case there were 115 children and adults, and, once again, there was a complete absence of acne. Surely we can just write that off to "genetics" and move on, right? Well, not exactly, because members of the same ethnic group living in urban settings eating a Westernized diet do experience acne! Dr. Cordain's group suggested that a diet that keeps insulin and blood sugar stable was the common, acne-protecting thread between the two groups evaluated. Dr. Logan subsequently reviewed the study and published his own hypothesis in the *Archives of Dermatology* (2003) that the high omega 3 content of these isolated communities might also be an acne-protective factor. Dr. William Danby of Dartmouth University also communicated with the study authors and it was determined that the consumption of dairy products was near nil in these isolated communities. Indeed, it is reported that the Aché consider the idea of milk consumption to be abhorrent. It is also likely that a variety of colorful antioxidants within the diets of isolated communities is also playing a role. We will explore the details of the acne-protective diet as we move through the book.

There had been hints over the years that lifestyle changes to isolated, traditional communities, and dietary changes in particular, could increase the rates of acne. From South America to Africa, from the northern parts of the polar regions to the land of the rising sun, much lower rates of acne have been described among those who maintain a traditional diet and lifestyle. For example, Dr. Otto Schaefer, a medical doctor who spent three decades treating the Inuit in the northern reaches of Alberta, Canada, noted that as the Western dietary influences encroached on the previously isolated community, the rates of acne soared. He witnessed the changes to the complexions occurring in a relatively short period of time. Dr. Schaefer recounted his first two decades of treating and working with the Inuit in the journal *Nutrition Today* (1971), where he stated, "Another condition has become prevalent, one obvious even to the layman: acne vulgaris." The traditional diet had consisted of fish, wild game, berries, roots, some greens, and seaweed. This, of course, would change in just a few short years—relative intakes of quality protein and complex carbohydrates would decline, while the sugar intake per person increased by 75 percent between 1959 and 1967.

Others had also taken notice of the situation in the northern polar regions. As medical journalist Elmer Bendiner stated in an article in the journal *Hospital Practice* (1974), "Acne vulgaris now scars the hitherto renowned complexions of the Eskimo and the evidence leaps at once from even the most casual glance at the faces of the youngsters who seem to be constantly nibbling at candy bars or drinking soda pop out of a can." We look upon it as slowly spreading smallpox carried in by Westerners when they infiltrate the traditional diets. Elmer Bendiner was obviously touched by this also in his polar experience in 1974 when he wrote, "Indeed the whites have swamped the Eskimo in a mass of sugar and carbohydrates."

Other doctors were reporting similar findings, including a complete absence of acne in those living in the Japanese island of Okinawa before it became Westernized. Now that the Okinawans have become the largest consumers of fast food within Japan, and the Okinawan men have fallen out of the number one spot in Japanese longevity, it would be interesting to see if acne has increased as the waistlines have expanded. We do know that the rates of acne in Japan have increased overall in the last thirty years—probably as a result of the changing Japanese diet. In 1964, Dr. Harumi Terada of the University of Tokyo, Faculty of Medicine, reported that extensive acne was much more common among young Americans versus their counterparts living in Tokyo and Yokohama. Japanese teens were about half as likely to have acne as the teens living in U.S. cities—and this wasn't a tiny study; there were about five hundred subjects examined in each country. Couldn't it be just genetics? Probably not, because new research in the *Japanese Journal of Dermatology* (2001) shows that the rates are now very high and similar to Westernized nations. Later, we will talk extensively about the acne-protective components of the traditional Japanese diet.

Researchers from Peru reported in the *Journal of Adolescent Health* (1998) that rates of acne were much lower in Peruvian Indians, actually close to 40 percent lower, than in whites living in Peru. Once again, this might be written off to genetics. However, they also made note that white teens in Peru were much less likely to have acne than their counterparts of the same age living in the United Kingdom. Perhaps some of the local dietary habits and lifestyle were influencing the acne rates among the whites of Arequipa, Peru.

Another diet-acne connection came to light when researchers from Portugal were trying to determine the prevalence of acne in northern Portugal. The study, published in the *Journal of the European Academy of Dermatology and Venereology* (2006), looked at some of the differences between the young students who had acne compared to those who did not have acne. Two differences emerged in the subjects with acne when compared to those without, and both of these differences were statistically significant—those with acne were more likely to consume soft drinks and chocolates.

Now let's talk about the second new study that opened the door to a fresh look at the acne-diet connection. This one was from the Harvard School of Public Health, and the results, published in the *Journal of the American Academy of Dermatology* (2005), also have some historical background. What these researchers found was a connection that had been batted around for decades by a few dermatologists— dairy consumption, and milk in particular, is associated with acne. Now while that is not positive news for the great state of Wisconsin, where the license plates are emblazoned with *America's Dairyland*, the research is in complete support of what has been reported over the last half century. A study published in the *Southern Medical Journal* (1949) had linked milk consumption with acne when almost two thousand patients kept strict food diaries. Dermatologist Dr. William Kaufman of Roanoke Memorial Hospital in Virginia reported in the *Medical Times* (1965), "It is difficult to escape the clinical impression that excessive milk drinking is involved in the causation of acne." Then in 1966, dermatologist Jerome Fisher presented his research at the annual meeting of the American Dermatological Association, research based on more than one thousand patients followed over a decade. His conclusion—milk is a principal villain when it comes to acne. A discussion of his research even made the pages of *Time* magazine (April 29, 1966) where it was stated that "Dr. Fisher advises teen-agers to cut down on foods rich in both fats and sweets—fried foods, ice cream, peanut butter, whole-milk cheeses, nuts and pastries." The man was way ahead of his time; he also noted the stress connection with acne in the interview, a connection that now has the support of published research and one we will explore later.

One of the criticisms of the Harvard acne-milk study was that it relied upon retrospective data—in other words, the participants were asked to recall the components of a high school diet from years before, and this was tied to reports of severe acne. To overcome retrospective reporting, it helps to have a huge study, and in this case it was with almost fifty thousand subjects as part of the Nurses Health Study II. To silence the critics, the Harvard researchers looked again, except this time in a prospective fashion—they knew what the diet was at baseline, with no recall required. They looked at data provided by more than six thousand girls ages nine to fifteen in 1996 and followed up in 1999 by presenting questionnaires concerning the presence and severity of acne to the same girls. Sure enough, the follow-up study published in the *Dermatology Online Journal* (2006) showed the same relationship between greater milk consumption and the occurrence of acne! The researchers theorize, as Dr. Fisher had done exactly forty years before, that milk promotes acne through a hormonal effect. At this point the researchers are unsure if milk promotes acne because of the growth hormones, reproductive hormones, and/or the many other growth factors it contains, or because of how it influences the release of our own growth hormones. It may be no coincidence that at least four precursors to DHEA (the "acne hormone") are present in milk from pregnant cows—about 85 percent of the milk we consume.

High-glycemic-index (GI) foods can spike blood sugar and lead to consistently high levels of insulin, the body's hormone sent out to get blood sugar into our cells. Although milk is technically a low-GI beverage, for reasons that are not entirely clear, it can markedly increase insulin levels. Research published in the *European Journal of Clinical Nutrition* (2001) shows that even small amounts of milk combined with other foods at a meal can spike insulin release. Interestingly, yogurt (which has not been connected to acne) has been shown to lower the expected rise in insulin release after consumption of test meals under experimental circumstances. The fermentation process may positively alter the proteins or carbohydrates that otherwise spike blood insulin.

We will explore this insulin-acne connection and dietary influences on the hormonal triggers of acne in the coming pages.

The Blockbuster

With this exciting new research focused on large population studies, Drs. Danby and Cordain and other cutting-edge researchers had lit the fuse for the Big One—the long-awaited controlled clinical trial. This was the logical and very necessary next step, a research design that would examine elements of the diet in a proper, controlled fashion. Dr. Neil Mann and colleagues from the Royal Melbourne Hospital in Australia took up the challenge and designed a trial that would be the first to examine the acne-diet connection under acceptable, modern scientific parameters. The results, published in the *Journal of the American Academy of Dermatology* (2007) would finally undo the unfair dismissal of a diet-acne connection—a long-held denial that was based more on thirty-year-old pseudoscience and less on credible research. Specifically, the Australian researchers set up a three-month trial where patients with acne were assigned to a controlled diet: low in simple carbohydrates, higher in fiber and protein, higher in polyunsaturated fat, and lower in saturated fats. The diet was described as a high protein and low glycemic load diet. We will discuss glycemic load in more detail in the hormone chapter; for now it is enough to know that the carbohydrates that were consumed were much less likely to spike blood sugar and insulin, and were more likely to include dietary fiber. The dietary intervention groups were advised to consume lean meats, poultry, fish, whole grains, and whole fruits. So as not to bias the participants in terms of acne, all were informed that the purpose of the study was to compare the carbohydrate to protein ratio in the diet and were not informed of the study's hypothesis related to acne. After twelve weeks, those in the high fiber, high protein diet group had total lesion counts that were significantly less than the control group. The dietary intervention group also had reduced weight, reduced levels of acne-promoting androgens, and more of the insulin-like growth factor binding protein that can hold onto the hormones and prevent them from causing acne. At the beginning of the study, these hormonal markers and the severity of acne were similar in both groups! Note the three-month time-frame the researchers used in the design of the study—it takes time for acne lesions (comedones) to both develop and heal through diet and lifestyle. We make this point now, and will do so again when we discuss the specifics of the Clear Skin Lifestyle to underscore the need for patience and commitment in the prevention and healing process.

A New Direction

The four new studies on a diet-acne connection are finally leading us down the right path. The floodgates are opened now, and indeed as we go to press with this book, we are informed that another acne-diet trial is soon to be published with similar results. Does that matter in acne? For most, you bet it does! Yes, acne is a complex condition influenced by many variables; however, why should it be any different from other complex chronic medical conditions that are, at least in part, mediated by diet? From diabetes to depression, from Alzheimer's disease to schizophrenia, researchers are uncovering nutritional connections to our most complicated diseases—and neither is acne immune to dietary influences. The new studies are only the beginning; they are just scratching the surface of potential mechanisms behind dietary influences on the genetics of acne. Now let's turn our attention to the inflammation and oxidative stress that are part of the acne process and examine how we can affect that cycle through dietary means.

Chapter Key Points

✔ Nutritional medicine is a new and emerging discipline.

✔ To date, the nutritional training of medical doctors has been very limited.

✔ The diet-acne connection was refuted in the 1970s by poorly designed studies no longer considered valid.

✔ There has been a shift toward pharmaco-dermatology as the pharmaceutical industry and its influence have grown.

✔ Nutritional training aside, dermatologists are the experts in the evaluation and treatment of skin conditions. Consultation is strongly recommended.

✔ Diet and lifestyle modifications work best when used in conjunction with conventional treatment.

✔ Some "acne mimics" can look like acne yet require differing treatment approaches—proper evaluation of skin conditions ensures health and safety.

✔ Chocolate comes in many forms; some can increase inflammation and oxidative stress while cocoa can do the opposite.

✔ While iodine may cause an acnelike condition, those who eat more fish and seafood tend to have less acne.

✔ Milk consumption is strongly associated with acne.

✔ Studies of global traditional diets (New Guinea, Paraguay, northern Canada, Okinawa) show a worsening of acne with the encroachment and influence of Western dietary habits.

3

Putting Out the Flames of Acne

VOLUMES AND VOLUMES OF INTERNATIONAL research have made it
very clear that inflammation is connected to virtually all chronic
health conditions, including heart disease, diabetes, obesity, cancer,
and, yes, even acne. Inflammation has gained celebrity status, recently
making the cover of *Time* magazine (February 23, 2004), where it
was referred to as "The Secret Killer." Indeed, chronic inflammation
wreaks havoc throughout the body, and our old friend the pilosebaceous unit is not exempt from the ravages of inflammation. This is a
more subtle, or low-grade inflammation, and not the high-end version
associated with the "itis" conditions like rheumatoid arthritis. Still, in
acne it is noticeable, so when you see marked redness surrounding an
acne lesion, or the red bump of a cystic acne lesion, you can be assured
that the fires of inflammation are burning. What we have in acne is, in
truth, a folliculitis, or an inflammation of the follicle. While much has
been written about the sebaceous gland, it is involved in a secondary
fashion. It is the inflammation directed at the foreign contents of the
follicle that fuels the flames of acne and its folliculitis.

Another feature of most chronic medical conditions is oxidative
stress, or free-radical damage. You can think of free radicals as bandits
that steal electrons from other molecules. The thievery process (loss
of electrons) is called oxidation, and it causes damage and promotes

further inflammation inside the pilosebaceous unit. However, our skin cells and pilosebaceous units have a pretty solid security operation known as the antioxidant defense system, which keeps unruly free radicals in check. This antioxidant defense system is perfectly designed to defend us against free-radical offenders and also prevent their formation. There is, however, one very important feature of the defense system related to nutritional medicine—our defense against free radicals is critically dependent upon dietary sources of antioxidants. Some major antioxidants are manufactured inside cells, but even here they require dietary nutrients to build them and make them effective.

With a colorful diet rich in fruits, vegetables, nuts, and culinary herbs, the antioxidant defense system works like a charm. Problems arise, however, when the production of free radicals exceeds the capacity of the defense system, or when the defense system is not supported by high-quality dietary fuel. More on antioxidants in a moment, but first let's turn to a more detailed look at inflammation in acne and how diet can make a difference.

Why Is Inflammation the Plague of the Twenty-first Century?

As you might imagine, the Western diet, with its hydrogenated trans and saturated fats, and its sedentary context, is the biggest contributor to the inflammation plague. Lack of dietary antioxidants has also been shown to promote inflammation, and, in turn, a state of chronic inflammation uses up precious antioxidants. To compound matters, psychological stress turns on inflammatory fires that help inflammation and free-radical generation to burn brightly.

Chronic inflammation is provoked by the excess intake of saturated fats and dietary sugars. In addition, our overconsumption of omega-6 fatty acids (e.g., corn, safflower, soybean, and sunflower oils) has been shown in many studies to promote inflammation. Together, the saturated fats, trans fats, and excess omega-6 fatty acids encourage the production of inflammatory chemicals called prostaglandins, particularly the series 2 type called PGE2; and leukotrienes, particularly a nasty one called LTB4. As we will see, both PGE2 and LTB4 are directly involved in acne. Now, as with our request regarding "pilosebaceous unit," please say "PGE2" and "LTB4" ten times quickly, and simply remember that they are inflammatory chemicals. These undesirable fats also direct the production of immune chemicals called *cytokines*, which also contribute to inflammation and the acne process. On the other hand, the omega-3 fatty acids have natural anti-inflammatory properties and are well known to dampen the inflammatory cascade. Fish, particularly oily ocean fish such as salmon, sardines, mackerel, and anchovies, is the most potent anti-inflammatory food you can put into your body because fish contains omega-3 fatty acids that diminish the activity of LTB4, PGE2, and the inflammatory cytokines. Canola oil, walnuts, deep green leafy vegetables, blueberries, and ground flaxseeds are also important sources of the anti-inflammatory omega-3 fatty acid.

The human genetic profile has remained constant over the past forty thousand years; however, the composition of our dietary fat intake has changed radically in the last half century. We have significantly increased our saturated and trans fat intake, while at the same time our consumption of precious omega-3 fatty acids has taken a serious plunge. The void of omega-3 is being filled by omega-6-rich corn, safflower, sunflower, and soybean oils. Omega-6 fats have found their way into our food supply at an excessive rate. Genetically we have been accustomed to an omega-6 to omega-3 ratio of close to 1:1, a far cry from the current ratio, which is at least ten parts, and up to twenty parts omega-6 for every one of omega-3. One common aspect of the traditional diets of those who are (or have been) relatively free of acne is a much greater intake of omega-3 fatty acids. Consider that the diet top-heavy in omega-6 oils promotes inflammation and oxidative stress, both of which contribute to the acne process. Excess saturated fats, and any amount of trans fat, can promote inflammation throughout the body, including within the pilosebaceous unit. Depending on your genetics, lifestyle, and environmental influences, a deficiency in omega-3 or an excess of other fats may promote acne and lengthen its recovery time.

As far back as 1967, researchers had documented the benefits of chemically reducing the production of LTB4 and PGE2 in acne. It has been forty years since distinguished dermatologist Dr. John Strauss and colleagues found that ETYA, a synthetic drug that inhibits the formation of LTB4 and PGE2, improved the appearance of acne and reduced the amount of sebum released into the follicle. Then, in the 1970s, a series of studies showed that zinc levels are low in acne patients, particularly those with more severe acne, and that oral zinc supplementation was helpful in the treatment of acne. The exact mechanisms behind the benefits of zinc in acne were far from completely understood, in fact, they really weren't understood at all. However, in the United Kingdom, a famed nutritional medicine expert and his young PhD student did have some clues for the benefits of zinc. In a brief commentary published in the *Archives of Dermatology* (1979), Dr. David Horrobin, an Oxford University–trained medical doctor, and his colleague, Stephen Cunnane, made the right connections between zinc, essential fatty acids, and inflammation in acne. They described treatment success with a combination of zinc sulfate and evening primrose oil in acne—the reason for the improvements was reported to be the synergistic anti-inflammatory effect of both zinc and essential fatty acids. This minor report had huge implications and would later open the door to further study of both widespread and local inflammation in acne, as well as nutritional interventions to curb the process. Since this report there have been numerous studies showing the anti-inflammatory and anti-oxidant effects of zinc.

The relationship between inflammation and acne had obviously sparked the interest of dermatologist Dr. V. M. Kovalev as he began investigating the blood levels of the inflammatory chemical PGE2 in acne patients. After demonstrating that PGE2 was elevated in thousands of assessments among acne patients, he performed a trial in 1982 with an oral anti-inflammatory drug. He reported significant improvements in more than 90 percent of the 104 acne patients in that group. The following year he published yet another study, which showed that the blood and skin levels of PGE2 were significantly correlated to all forms of acne. What he did not know in 1982–83, which we now know, was that omega-3–rich fish oil, and the eicosapentaenoic acid (EPA) omega-3 in particular, can significantly reduce PGE2 in humans at just a few grams per day—without the side effects of some prescription nonsteroidal anti-inflammatory drugs. We also now know that overconsumption of omega-6–rich linoleic acid oils (corn, safflower, sunflower, soybean) can easily promote the production of PGE2.

One might imagine that the work of the good doctor Kovalev would have spurred further investigation of the role of anti-inflammatory medications in acne—however, since Dr. Kovalev was from the former Soviet Union and the studies were published in Russian journals, no one picked up on them. Instead, mainstream research continued to focus on the anti-inflammatory effects of existing therapies, including antibiotics. The focus centered on the *P. acnes*, the bacterium we talked about that can promote the production of inflammatory chemicals within the pilosebaceous unit. It was also assumed that the inflammation of acne, as bad as it might be, was only a secondary feature of the work of *P. acnes*—we now know better. Unlike Dr. Kovalev, few were thinking about investigating more widespread inflammation or decreasing the acne inflammation cascade from the inside out.

There were a few exceptions, and a tiny sprinkling of case reports and small studies over the years suggested that oral anti-inflammatory medications, including ibuprofen, might improve outcome when added to mainstream therapies. These findings, including the original report in 1967 that the chemical inhibition of LTB4 and PGE2 can improve acne and lower sebum production, were not lost on Dr. Hal Schaffer, a dermatologist working at the University of Michigan School of Medicine. He immediately recognized the potential value of fish oils rich in EPA and DHA in lowering LTB4 and PGE2, and in the *International Journal of Dermatology* (1989), he called for a controlled study of omega-3 fatty acids to be conducted in acne. One suspects that if fish oils could have been patented, the pharmaceutical industry would have championed their cause twenty years ago. In any case, the potential of anti-inflammatory medications and supplements in acne was not a hotbed of research, and things were once again silent for another decade.

Finally, in 2001 Dr. Christos C. Zouboulis of the University of Berlin and colleagues reported on some remarkable findings that were very reminiscent of Dr. Kovalev's work and Dr. Strauss's before him. Rather than focusing on PGE2, the German researchers examined the other inflammatory chemical called LTB4, also thought to be involved in promoting inflammation within the pilosebaceous unit by a number of mechanisms. The manufacture of LTB4 is highly dependent upon dietary factors, including the linoleic acid found in corn, safflower, sunflower, and soybean oils. Dietary linoleic acid within these oils is converted into arachidonic acid, and in excess this arachidonic acid can be a nasty creature that in turn promotes the manufacture of both LTB4 and PGE2—two different pathways with one common result—inflammation.

Dr. Zouboulis and colleagues decided to have a look at a medication called zileuton (Zyflo), which is well known to prevent the conversion of arachidonic acid into LTB4. The results, formally reported in the *Archives of Dermatology* (2003), were more than remarkable. There was a 71 percent reduction in inflammatory acne lesions after twelve weeks, and the overall reduction in severity was reported to be 59 percent. The photographic evidence printed along with the results is certainly impressive. Since zileuton has no documented antibacterial activities, the results strongly suggest that we don't need antibiotics to dampen inflammatory pathways, and they also suggest that inflammation is not merely a minor player involved due to increased bacteria. As recently pointed out in the most detailed review of acne and inflammation, published in *Clinics in Dermatology* (2004), it now appears that inflammatory events "may be the earliest events in acne lesion formation." While the bacteria *P. acnes* may be a player in the development of an acne lesion, including promoting further inflammation, it is by no means the only player. Another is the yeast *Malassezia*, which is present in 68 percent of acne papules. It is well known to induce severe itching and pustular inflammation in one of acne's major mimics, *Malassezia* folliculitis. Inflammation may be occurring throughout the entire acne process, with or without *P. acnes.*

Since the initial clinical work that documented the benefits of zileuton, Dr. Zouboulis's group has performed more detailed investigations on why blocking LTB4 might be helpful in acne. Writing in the journal *Dermatology* (2005), they reported that oral zileuton can directly reduce the amount of sebum manufactured by the sebaceous gland—a finding Dr. Strauss had reported almost forty years earlier. Remember our discussion in the first chapter of how the overproduction of sebum is a central feature to acne development? It was shown that zileuton reduced sebum production to levels similar to the wonder drug isotretinoin (Accutane). Then in the *Journal of Molecular*

Medicine (2006), the doors were blown wide open by showing for the first time that the sebocytes, the cells that make up our oil-producing sebaceous glands, can actually manufacture PGE2 and LTB4 from arachidonic acid. So now we know that the oral administration of agents that are capable of preventing the conversion of arachidonic acid into these inflammatory chemicals (PGE2 and LTB4) is reducing inflammation and preventing the buildup of sebum right at the level of the pilosebaceous unit.

Further support to this entire acne-inflammation theory comes from a recent report in the European journal *Acta Dermato-Veneologica* (2006), where researchers documented significant improvements in severe acne with Enbrel, a drug that interferes with inflammatory cytokine production. Specifically, the medication targets TNFα, a cytokine involved in arthritis. Knowing that TNFα and other cytokines are also involved in acne, the Italian dermatologists decided to give the drug a go, even though the case did not involve arthritis. They reported significant improvements over twelve weeks, and almost complete regression after twenty-four weeks. The twenty-two-year-old patient had previously tried virtually all topical and oral medications without response.

All of this is well and good, and you're probably beginning to think that we are sales reps for zileuton at this point. While we wish the makers of zileuton well, we see this research from a totally different perspective—our view is from the vantage point of nutritional medicine. Patents have now been placed on the use of zileuton and various other prescription drugs for the treatment of inflammatory acne. Based on detailed experimental studies, it has been speculated that a potential prescription drug agent to treat inflammatory acne should be capable of blocking both PGE2 and LTB4. Yet, the most precious PGE2 and LTB4 inhibitor in nature is non-patentable fish oil, and in particular the eicosapentaenoic acid (EPA) omega-3 fatty acid. Higher omega-3 intake, as we have already discussed, represents a cornerstone of the low rates of acne among the traditional diets once found in Japan, the coastal regions of North Carolina, the Inuit of Canada, the Kitavan Islanders of Papua New Guinea and the Aché community of Paraguay. There is a wealth of research showing that EPA can reduce PGE2, LTB4, and the cytokine TNFα. There are lots of animal and human studies that show fish oil rich in EPA can improve inflammation in many conditions, perhaps most notably arthritis and cardiovascular disease. When it comes to supplementation, it takes about 2 grams of EPA to get the desired clinical interference with the inflammation cascade and reduced production of the inflammatory cytokines LTB4 and PGE2.

Fish oil has also been combined with other anti-inflammatory oils and ingredients to dampen inflammation. In fact, one study by Wake Forest University researchers published in the journal *Clinical Therapeutics* (2003) showed that a combination of EPA and gamma-linolenic acid (GLA) could decrease LTB4 to the same level as could zileuton. Note that GLA is found in evening primrose oil, the anti-inflammatory fatty acid that Dr. David Horrobin had found to be helpful in acne more than two decades earlier. Administration of GLA from evening primrose, borage, and black-currant oils can also lower the PGE2 inflammatory pathway.

The research showing that the cells that make up our oil-producing sebaceous glands can actually manufacture PGE2 and LTB4 from arachidonic acid also provides a mechanism for vegetable oils' promotion of acne. This was something Dr. Logan was convinced of when he was fifteen years old back in the mid-1980s. He had no idea of the mechanisms back then, but after continuous self-experimentation he was convinced that tuna fish packed in vegetable oil would lead to acne flare-ups—but not so with tuna packed in water. The overconsumption of our major dietary vegetable oils—corn, sunflower, safflower, soybean—is fanning the flames of acne by promoting production of arachidonic acid, which is the inflammatory fuel at the pilosebaceous unit. Saturated fats are not immune from the promotion of this inflammatory cascade. One saturated fat in particular, palmitic acid, which is found in high levels in palm oil, has been shown to interfere with the enzyme that normally breaks down PGE2, therefore leaving more of it around to wreak havoc. Many acne patients have complained about tropical oil such as palm oil in foods as being an acne-promoter.

Along the way, a major stumbling block to the pursuit of this line of research in acne arose: that certain vegetable oils might actually promote acne (a few studies that examined the fatty acid content of the sebum from acne lesions in patients with acne found much lower

Various Sources of EPA and DHA

Fish/Seafood	Total EPA/DHA (mg/100 g)
mackerel	2,300
chinook salmon	1,900
herring	1,700
anchovy	1,400
sardine	1,400
coho salmon	1,200
trout	600
spiny lobster	500
halibut	400
shrimp	300
catfish	300
sole	200
cod	200

levels of linoleic acid compared to non-acne controls). Many in the dermatology community took this to mean that low levels of linoleic acid must be a causative factor, so the obvious answer was, "Let's give more linoleic acid," which means, "Let's give more vegetable oils!" Thanks to recent advances, we finally have a very plausible reason for the low levels of linoleic acid in the sebum of acne patients—and the answer does not provide a reason to give more vegetable oils. We now know that linoleic acid is being more rapidly converted into arachidonic acid, then this arachidonic acid, in turn, is converted into PGE2 and LTB4, which promote inflammation. The low levels of

Omega-6 and Omega-3 Content (Percent) of Dietary Oils

Oil	Omega-6	Omega-3
safflower	75	0
sunflower	65	0
corn	54	0
cottonseed	50	0
sesame	42	0
peanut	32	0
soybean	51	7
canola	20	9
walnut	52	10
flax	14	57

Acne Nutrient Highlight—Eicosapentaenoic Acid

What is it?

Eicosapentaenoic Acid (EPA) is an important omega-3 fatty acid found in fish and seafood, particularly oily, ocean fish such as sardines, mackerel, and anchovies.

Why is it of value?

EPA is arguably the greatest anti-inflammatory found in nature. It reduces the production of two major acne-related chemicals— PGE2 and LTB4. It also lowers inflammatory cytokines, which are implicated in acne. In addition, human studies show a mood-regulating effect of EPA, and it may assist with resilience to the stress-related promotion of acne.

---

linoleic acid inside the sebum are almost certainly a consequence of the inflammatory cascade, so to suggest soybean oil (or any other oil rich in linoleic acid) as a means to combat acne would be like trying to put out a California wildfire by dumping kerosene from the sky instead of water.

Let's turn our attention back to the traditional diets of the Aché and Kitavans, the folks insulated from the influences of the high-sugar Western diet. The dietary protection against acne had been rightly attributed by the researchers to the lack of foods that spike blood sugar and insulin release. However, being aware of the work of Dr. Zouboulis and the role of inflammation in acne, Dr. Logan theorized that the traditional diets of the Aché and Kitavans would be higher in anti-inflammatory omega-3 fatty acids. His hypothesis that a higher intake of omega-3 fatty acids among traditional diets might be protective in acne was published in the *Archives of Dermatology* (2003). In his follow-up commentary, Dr. Cordain's team did confirm that the diets of the Aché and Kitavans are indeed higher in omega-3 levels, and the overconsumption of the vegetable oils that promote LTB4 and PGE2 production is a nonissue for these groups.

Nicotinamide and Inflammation

A few scientists working in the dermatology field had taken notice of the anti-inflammatory properties of the B vitamin nicotinamide. In

1970 it was demonstrated that the vitamin is well absorbed through the skin after topical application, and since then it has been investigated for the improvement of skin appearance, wound healing, aging, and the prevention of UV sun damage. In 1995, researchers from the State University of New York conducted a very well-designed study—a head-to-head comparison of topical nicotinamide vs. the old dermatology standby of topical clindamycin (antibiotic). While the study cites both products as sharing a "comparable efficacy," the numbers looked better for the vitamin! Sadly, while topical antibiotics are still listed among the standard therapies for acne, topical nicotinamide is not, and today few dermatologists recommend this option.

The benefits of oral nicotinamide were considered, and reported anecdotally. In the *Archives of Dermatology* (1975), Polish dermatologist Dr. Stephania Jablonska reported solid results with oral nicotinamide added to standard acne therapies. The Polish dermatologic group had been using oral nicotinamide (1,000 mg) in combination with the B vitamin riboflavin (B2, 18 mg), with success for the better part of a decade. Although not always necessary, they found that adding 1,000 mg of vitamin C and 150 mg of vitamin B6 also added to the beneficial effects.

Sadly, the initial reports of nicotinamide success were not followed up, and like many nutritional interventions for acne, the work of Dr. Jablonska sat in the medical archive collecting dust. That changed recently when a large open study determined that the anti-inflammatory properties of nicotinamide may indeed work from the inside out. The Nicomide Improvement in Clinical Outcomes Study (NICOS) was reported in the journal *Cutis* (2006). Dr. Neil Niren of the University of Pittsburgh and Dr. Helen Torok examined the value of a nicotinamide, zinc, copper, and folic acid combo in 149 acne patients. Improvement was rated by participants as a percentage reduction in the number of pimples and/or pustules during the therapy. After four weeks of therapy, 82 percent of the acne patients rated the overall change as either moderately or much better. This figure increased to 88 percent at the conclusion of the two-month trial. There was a particular benefit in the reduction of inflammatory acne lesions. The authors also noted that the addition of oral antibiotic to the vitamin-mineral regimen did not increase the percentage of patients responding. In the study, Nicomide tablets were taken either once or twice a day—it is currently available as a prescription item from your dermatologist. As with zinc, it is interesting to note that nicotinamide is involved in the metabolism of essential fatty acids and has been shown to improve mental function and decrease anger and stress reactivity.

While Nicomide as an oral supplement is an interesting concept in the treatment of acne, we do have a few concerns. First and foremost is the 50 mg of zinc oxide found in two tablets—combine this with the typical 10 mg or more found in a multivitamin, and you might end up taking far too much zinc. Note that the National Academies of Sciences has set the tolerable upper limit of zinc at 40 mg—beyond this daily intake of zinc there may be issues with immune system dysfunction. Then there is the issue of the recommended dietary allowance (RDA) of food dyes—Nicomide provides a daily dose of Blue #1 and Yellow #6. While we are being facetious about the RDA for synthetic chemicals, in general we do recommend avoidance of artificial coloring agents. Moving on we will explore a number of other antiacne nutrients that were overlooked in the Nicomide formula.

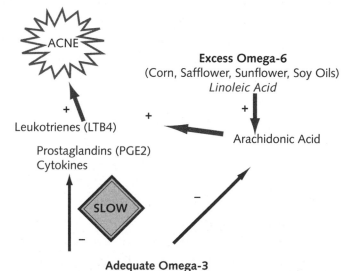

Oxidative Stress and Acne

There is another acne-protective aspect of the diet of the Aché, Kitavans, and other groups with minimal Western dietary influence—higher antioxidant intake. Traditional diets with an emphasis on colored-plant foods and seafood provide a host of antioxidant vitamins, minerals, and those critically important phytochemicals. The research story behind oxidative stress in acne is one that takes the same twists and turns as the inflammation connection. Once again, we have a few scientists and dermatologists who were way ahead of their time and working within the realm of non-patentable nutritional medicine. Once again they were basically unheeded by the profession at large.

In 1978, long before *antioxidant* would become a health buzzword, Drs. Samuel Ayers Jr. and Richard Mihan reported on successful acne treatment with a combination of oral vitamins A and E. At that time, vitamin A as a treatment for acne was not new; it had been around for quite some time, primarily to correct the overproduction of the cells lining the follicle channel. Yet what Dr. Ayers and Dr. Mihan were suggesting was an additional benefit and an entirely new concept. They were thinking about using vitamins A and E as fat-soluble antioxidants in an effort to limit the severity of acne—they were attempting to expand upon the work of Dr. Alloys L. Tappel, a food science professor at the University of California (Davis), who previously suggested that free radical damage and oxidative stress inside the follicle might be central to the acne process. Commenting in the *International Journal of Dermatology* (1978), Dr. Ayers and Dr. Mihan stated the synergistic combination of vitamins A and E was employed with a high degree of success and that "The new regimen has eliminated the necessity of antibiotics such as tetracycline, and we have virtually eliminated their use."

Remember our old friend Dr. V. M. Kovalev, the Russian dermatologist who was examining the role of anti-inflammatory medications in acne? You didn't think he was uninvolved in the free-radical/oxidative-stress story, did you? No, he was hard at work around the same time examining the role of antioxidants in the treatment of acne. In two separate studies published in 1981, he found that lipoic acid, one of the human body's most crucial antioxidants, was low in the blood of acne patients—in fact it was twice as low as those without acne. Alpha-lipoic acid is available in supplement form, and it is a valuable anti-oxidant because it works in both water and fat-soluble environments of the body. Decades after the work of Dr. V. M. Kovalev, lipoic acid would be included in virtually all high-end topical beauty products. His research suggested that lipoic acid was low due to standard treatments, including the antibiotics and other prescription medications. Dr. Kovalev found that the addition of alpha-lipoic acid improves treatment outcomes in acne and shortens the length of time required to get results from standard acne care.

Back in Los Angeles, Drs. Ayers and Mihan followed up with further reports on their protocol, which used high-dose water-soluble vitamin A (50,000 IU twice daily) and natural-source vitamin E (400 IU twice daily), combined with a low-sugar and low-fat diet. Writing in the journal *Cutis* (1981), the pair reported on ninety-eight patients prescribed the oral A-and-E combination along with a healthy diet, and, interestingly, the advice to drink no more than one glass of milk per day—these guys were clearly ahead of their time. It is also likely to be no coincidence that they practiced dermatology not far from Dr. Jerome Fisher, who had put the acne and milk connection on the map a few years earlier. This was not a controlled study; however, they did report that 90 percent of the patients had a good-to-excellent response, with marked improvements occurring after six to eight weeks. Please note that we are not advocating self-prescription of such high levels of vitamin A, as this requires close medical supervision.

Also in 1981, Drs. Kligman, Mills, and Leyden published an important paper called "Oral vitamin A in acne." While they did not tout the antioxidant value of the vitamin, they did state that oral retinol (vitamin A) has a "definite place in the treatment of serious acne." They provided step-by-step instructions to dermatologists on how to use oral vitamin A effectively and promised it would be the "first of many studies"—this, however, turned out not to be the case.

Sadly, the research presented on oral vitamin A was published on the eve of the grand North American unveiling of the vitamin A–like wonder drug Accutane, and the case for oral antioxidants once again went cold. There were some case reports published by Dr. S. R. Acharya of Mysore University in India, who found that oral vitamin E taken daily led to significant improvements among young adults (ages eighteen to twenty-two) with long-term acne. Things were, however, very quiet for vitamins A and E.

In 1990 Dr. Gerd Michaëlsson, a dermatologist from Uppsala, Sweden, reported some of her research on oxidative stress among acne patients in a European dermatology journal. She discovered that patients with inflammatory acne have significantly lower blood selenium levels than healthy controls without acne. Selenium plays a critical role in our antioxidant defense system, and a host of epidemiological studies link a lowered selenium status to cancer, neurodegenerative conditions, depression, and cardiovascular disease. Selenium has been shown to be particularly important in chronic inflammatory conditions where the oxidative stress burden is high. While her U.S. counterparts Drs. Ayers and Mihan were experimenting with vitamins A and E, Dr. Michaëlsson was reporting excellent results from her preliminary studies with selenium and vitamin E. Interestingly, a study in the *European Journal of Clinical Nutrition* (2003) involving almost fifteen thousand U.S. adults showed that higher levels of the inflammatory marker C-reactive protein are associated with low blood levels of vitamin A, selenium, and lycopene (an antioxidant carotenoid)—so the benefits of antioxidant vitamins in acne may involve their ability to cut off the inflammatory cycle. Lycopene is an important antioxidant from tomatoes that may also influence the hormonal aspects of acne—we will discuss this nutrient in greater detail later.

The potential of oral antioxidants received relatively little attention until 2005, and then things really gathered momentum. In three separate studies from different laboratories in Turkey, it was shown that the levels of the enzymes that control the antioxidant defense system are altered in acne. The enzymes are the machinery that allows the antioxidant defense system to function, and they are highly dependent upon nutrients such as selenium in order to perform at optimal levels. You can think of enzymes as a key turning on an ignition and starting the engine. Writing in the journal *Acta Dermatoven* (2005), the researchers stated, "Our findings show that drugs with antioxidant effects may be valuable in acne."

As interesting as these enzyme studies are, and they clearly show a

Fish and Seafood—Clearing Up the Controversy

Preliminary studies have shown that the highest consumers of fish and seafood have the lowest rates of acne, and those with acne are twice as likely to consume no fish at all. In *The Clear Skin Diet,* we provide the anti-inflammatory pathways that make the omega-3 fatty acids in fish and seafood a prime candidate for acne protection. Since we advocate fish consumption, it is important to clear up the controversy and widespread misinformation that exists in books and Internet sources.

1. *What are the best sources of omega-3 fatty acids?* Oily fish including salmon, sardines, anchovies, and mackerel are very high in the anti-inflammatory omega-3 fats called EPA and DHA. Most fish and seafood, even freshwater sources, do contain some level of omega-3 fatty acids.

2. *Are these fish safe? Aren't they high in mercury?* None of these fish are high in mercury. Contrary to popular opinion, the mercury in both farmed and wild salmon is negligible. Farmed salmon is, however, high in toxic environmental chemicals called polychlorinated biphenyl compounds (PCBs), which have been linked to cancer and cognitive dysfunction. You don't need to shop at high-end gourmet shops to buy wild salmon. Most canned salmon is in fact wild Canadian and Alaskan salmon—check the label for the wild source logo.

3. *So which fish are high in mercury?* Fresh tuna sushi/sashimi, tuna steaks, swordfish, shark, and tilefish are at the top of the list. However, new FDA data suggest that grouper, sea trout, orange

potential for antioxidant nutrients in acne, it was an even more recent study by a group from Jordan University of Science and Technology that finally put antioxidants on the acne map. These researchers measured the blood levels of vitamins A and E among one hundred patients newly diagnosed (and untreated) with acne—using drug-free patients is a good thing in research because then we know the measurements will not be confounded by medications. The results, published in *Clinical and Experimental Dermatology* (2006), showed that the patients with acne had significantly lower levels of vitamins A and E, and here is where it gets good—the lower the levels of vitamins A and E, the more severe roughy, and bluefish are all of concern. When it comes to canned tuna, the more expensive version, white albacore, has higher levels of mercury than previously thought. The chunk light is low in mercury and more acceptable for regular consumption. For more details and a tuna calculator based on weight and gender, see the Environmental Working Group resource at www.ewg.org.

4. *Is salmon a source of the linoleic acid we are currently overconsuming?* Only farmed salmon contains significant amounts of the linoleic acid that can drive inflammation. Linoleic acid is virtually absent from wild sources.

5. *Is it possible to reduce environmental toxins through cooking?* Research has shown that up to 50 percent of PCBs can be reduced through various cooking methods and with removal of the skin from fish. Unfortunately, the opposite is true of mercury. With cooking, the mercury remains behind, leading to concentrations per weight that are 45 percent higher than raw fish. It is even worse when fish are breaded and fried in oil—here the mercury levels are more than 70 percent higher than raw fish.

6. *In the final analysis, do the benefits of fish intake outweigh the risks?* Yes! After extensive review, researchers from Harvard's School of Public Health reported in the *Journal of the American Medical Association* (2006) that the benefits of fish intake do exceed the potential risks. The researchers advised sidestepping the high-mercury fish and including a wide variety of fish and seafood to minimize risk.

the acne. With one hundred patients with acne and one hundred age-matched control subjects, the study was certainly large enough to provide meaningful results and was a step up from the old study of four or five people who didn't get worse from eating chocolate. It is likely that the blood levels of antioxidants are used up more readily in those with acne because there is a greater demand to deal with free radicals—this is actually a common occurrence in chronic medical conditions characterized by both oxidative stress and inflammation. It was also of note that even though the researchers well-matched the acne patients with one hundred healthy controls of the same age, the dietary assessments revealed that the acne patients were less likely to consume fruits and vegetables and more likely to eat carbohydrates and fast foods! Therefore, it is also possible that acne patients consume less antioxidant-rich foods than do young adults without acne.

Some nineteen years earlier, Dr. Demetre Labadarios and colleagues had also reported that patients with acne have much lower blood levels of vitamin A. Writing in the journal *Clinical and Experimental Dermatology* (1987), they reported on the dietary differences that might account for the lower levels of vitamin A. Wouldn't you know it, the patients with acne were less-frequent consumers of green leafy vegetables and fruit. One other interesting note came out of this study—acne patients were also less-frequent consumers of fish! Compared to the age-matched healthy control group drawn from the same university, the acne patients were twice as likely to consume no fish at all. The healthy controls were twice as likely to consume fruit every day and four times as likely versus acne patients to consume green leafy vegetables every day . Beyond the moderate levels of vitamin A found in some fish, the arrows were once again pointing to an omega-3–acne-prevention connection. The researchers just didn't know it at the time.

When it comes to vitamin E supplementation for human skin conditions, it is comforting to know that oral vitamin E does make its way to the skin surface. In fact, oral vitamin E becomes incorporated right into the oily sebum itself. Interestingly, although research published in the *Annals of the New York Academy of Sciences* (2004) shows that blood levels of vitamin E rise quickly after oral supplementation, such is not the case in the skin. Evaluation shows that it actually takes about three weeks before oral vitamin E levels translate into significant elevations in the sebum. This makes sense when you consider that the fat-manufacturing cell of the pore (the sebocyte) takes about two weeks to grow from its immature state to a fully formed fat-filled cell that ruptures and bursts its contents into the follicle.

Smoke Equals Fire

Further support for the free-radical theory of acne comes from the examination of adults who are smokers. Anecdotally, it had been

---

Acne Nutrient Highlight—Zinc

What is it?

Zinc is an essential mineral involved in more than three hundred different enzyme reactions, so it's not surprising that zinc has a hand in many biological pots within the body—important roles have been documents in growth and development, brain function, immune function, and reproduction, to name a few. Zinc can be found in oysters, lean meats, beans, nuts, seeds, oatmeal, whole grains, and Japanese miso.

Why is it of value?

While the precise mechanisms of zinc's benefits in acne are not understood, we know that it acts as an important antioxidant and anti-inflammatory nutrient for the skin. It is also involved in the metabolism of omega-3 fatty acids. Zinc is responsible for releasing and transporting the antiacne nutrient vitamin A from liver storage. Zinc helps clear away and break down substance P, a nerve chemical that promotes sebum production under stress. Various studies over the last three decades have shown that zinc levels are lower in acne patients than healthy controls, and that oral and/or topical zinc supplementation may be of therapeutic value. Studies also show that zinc may be of value in protecting against depression.

---

reported by some clinicians that there may be a connection between the two; however, it was only in 2001 when the issue was given proper research attention. Dr. Torsten Schafer and colleagues from the University of Munich examined the better part of one thousand citizens of Hamburg, and what they found was that overall, acne was more prevalent in smokers. More specifically, the results, published in the *British Journal of Dermatology* (2001), showed a very strong relationship between the number of cigarettes smoked and the severity of acne—this is referred to as a dose-dependent relationship. Dr. Schafer's group didn't speculate too much on possible mechanisms behind the acne-smoking relationship. It has been shown that smokers have higher levels of free testosterone, and the more you smoke, the higher the testosterone. As highlighted in the *International Journal of*

Feed Your Skin

The highest antioxidant-rich foods include:

acai	cilantro	oregano
alfalfa	cinnamon	parsley
apple sauce	cloves	peaches
apple vinegar	cocoa	pears
artichoke	cranberry	plums
asparagus	dates	pomegranate
avocado	eggplant	prunes
basil	elderberry	purple cauliflower
beans (red, pinto, black, navy)	figs	purple sweet potato
	Fuji apples	raspberry
beets	ginger	red cabbage
bell peppers	green tea	red grapes
black-eyed peas	high-quality olive oil	red leaf lettuce
black pepper	kale	red potatoes
blackberry	nuts (all are high, wal-	spinach
blueberry	nuts in particular)	strawberry
broccoli	oatmeal and *whole*	tangerines
Brussels sprouts	*grain* breakfast	turmeric
cherries	cereals	
chili powder	oranges	

Andrology (2006), smokers have 15 percent higher total testosterone, and 13 percent higher free, or active, testosterone. It could also be that more than a few acne patients turn to cigarettes in an attempt to alleviate the stress of acne itself. However, allow us to indulge in one other possible mechanism—increased oxidative stress. It is well known that smokers are under increased oxidative stress, generate more free radicals, and have lower blood levels of important antioxidant nutrients. Why? Because they need more of these vital antioxidants and use them up more readily in defense of the body. Knowing what we know now about free radicals and antioxidant nutrients in acne, it is more than plausible that smoking may contribute to acne because it lowers the antioxidant defenses, promotes inflammatory chemical production, and, to top it all off, it can interfere with the metabolism of omega-3 fatty acids.

The Anti-Inflammatory/Antioxidant Foods

When it comes to reducing inflammation and providing an anti-oxidant punch, certain foods do stand out from the rest. While these nutritional powerhouses can make a difference to most people, individual sensitivities and allergies are always possible. The bottom line is, all foods are not the ideal for each person.

FISH OIL

This is perhaps the greatest natural anti-inflammatory substance found in the diet. There are now volumes of international research

---

Acne Nutrient Highlight—Vitamin A

What is it?

Vitamin A belongs to a class of compounds called retinoids. The active alcohol form of vitamin A is known as retinol and is referred to as preformed vitamin A. Beta-carotene and other "carotenoids" are referred to as pro-vitamin A as they can be converted in the human body into retinol. Vitamin A has many functions in the body, including the support of immune function, red blood cell production, healthy skin, normal vision, and growth and development. Vitamin A is an important antioxidant and low levels of this vitamin have been associated with inflammation and acne. Sources include sweet potatoes, cod liver oils, orange or yellow fruits and vegetables, spinach, and cod liver oil.

Why is it of value?

Oral and topical vitamin A has been used for years by dermatologists with success in treating acne. The precise mechanisms of action are not fully understood at this time. However, we do know that vitamin A is essential in the normal shedding of the cells that line the follicle walls. This, in turn, prevents a sticky or cohesive buildup of cells that would otherwise plug up the pore. In addition, it is likely that the antioxidant and anti-inflammatory properties of vitamin A are at work in promoting healthy skin. We recommend guidance from a healthcare provider when using more than the tolerable upper limit of 10,000 IU or 3000 micrograms of preformed vitamin A. Pregnant women should not go beyond 2600 IU or 800 micrograms per day unless directed by a healthcare provider.

that document the ability of omega-3 fatty acids, particularly the eicosapentaenoic acid (EPA) found in fish oil, to dampen the cascade of inflammation. In fact, the anti-inflammatory effect is so valuable, and the wealth of scientific evidence so strong, that an editorial in the *Journal of Rheumatology* (2000) stated, "Thus, the clinical data achieve the highest standard of proof of efficacy proposed for evidence based medicine (i.e., meta analysis of RCT). . . . Dietary fish oil supplements should now be regarded as part of standard therapy for rheumatoid arthritis." Seven years after this directive, the research has only become stronger for omega-3 fatty acids and the reduction of inflammation. Note that EPA is the primary anti-inflammatory component of fish oil and many supplements provide just a small amount of EPA. The guidelines for arthritis suggest at least 2,000 mg, while in acne we would suggest at least 1,000 mg of actual EPA (not just fish oil) daily. Check the labels and make sure your brand has enough EPA.

WHOLE GRAINS

Whole grains are a cornerstone to dampening inflammation, and they also provide much-needed antiacne nutrients and antioxidants. Researchers at Tufts University have reported that most whole grain or fiber-rich foods actually score very highly when it comes to antioxidant protection. Therefore, not only are we losing key nutrients when we strip away grains and peel off fiber through processing, we are also taking away valuable antioxidants. Whenever possible, choose whole grain breads, cereals and pasta. Logos such as "Contains Whole Grains," etc., do not make products automatic choices. Food companies know that *whole grains* is a buzzword these days, and they can easily meet the smidgen of whole grain required to make claims in a cereal-based product. As a consumer and acne patient, always check labels for two things when it comes to grain-containing products (e.g., breads and cereals): (1) How many grams of sugar are there? and (2) How many grams of fiber are there? The former number should be as low as possible, and the latter number should be as high as possible.

TURMERIC

Otherwise known as *Curcuma longa*, this is the yellow powder found in curry. There are a number of healthy chemicals within turmeric;

perhaps the best known is curcumin. This chemical has shown itself to be an incredible antioxidant with significant anti-inflammatory properties. At least four human studies have shown that curcumin can decrease inflammation, and a host of studies show that it can specifically inhibit the inflammation-promoting immune chemicals called cytokines.

GINGER

Since turmeric and ginger are in the same plant family, it should be no big shock that ginger would also have significant anti-inflammatory and antioxidant properties. Ginger has a 2,500-year history of traditional use in India and other parts of Asia as a medicinal agent. Much like turmeric, ginger has many active chemicals, and researchers have focused on gingerol for its medicinal properties. There is no question that ginger is an anti-inflammatory agent. Not only is this idea supported by animal studies, but also in at least four human studies as well. The gingerols have been shown to specifically inhibit inflammatory chemicals PGE2 and LTB4, which are of significance in acne.

Liberal use of ginger and turmeric is encouraged, as both should be considered bodyguards of the pilosebaceous unit, and both can put out the flames of inflammation.

GREEN TEA

Research shows that regular consumption of green tea has multiple health benefits. Green tea contains a blend of phytochemicals called catechins, which are potent antioxidants with significant anti-inflammatory properties. In particular, epigallocatechin-3-gallate (EGCG) is a key player among the catechins, and it is known to suppress the inflammatory chemicals called cytokines and prostaglandins that are involved in acne.

In the next chapter we will discuss the benefits of green tea on the hormonal aspects of acne. It is also of note that green tea inhibits the growth of potentially harmful bacteria, yet, incredibly, it promotes the growth of beneficial bacteria—*Lactobacillus* and *Bifidobacteria*—in the gastrointestinal tract. We will discuss that in greater detail in chapter 5. Recent human studies have also shown that green tea, and the antioxidant chemical EGCG in particular, can assist in the reduction of abdominal fat. There are a number of ways in which the accumulation of abdominal fat can contribute to the inflammation and oxidative stress cycle in acne—more on that later too.

Green tea has played a major role in the traditional Japanese diet for years. The highest grade of green tea is Japanese *matcha*—a fine powder of the finest green tea leaves that are grown in the shade. Researchers from the University of Colorado reported in 2003 that the concentration of EGCG available from drinking matcha is up to 137 times greater than the amount of EGCG available from other commercially available green teas. The powdered matcha has some advantages for someone who may not be a big tea drinker, because small amounts can also be incorporated into baked goods, smoothies, and desserts.

Experimental studies suggest that green tea may induce a deficiency of the B vitamin folic acid by its inhibition of an enzyme involved in folate metabolism. If you are drinking more than a couple of cups of green tea a day, or taking green tea supplements, then taking a folic acid supplement may be advisable.

NUTS

In general, nuts have been unfairly dismissed as a fat-laden dietary item that should be avoided. The tide is turning, and after some high-profile scientific research, nuts have emerged as a health food. We urge patients with acne to experiment with different nuts. The traditional clear skin diets of the 1950s and 1960s often excluded consumption of nuts, and peanuts in particular—however, we are not ready to write off all nuts so quickly. It is entirely possible that some nuts may cause breakouts, while others have no effect. The problem may be in the way the nuts are prepared. For some, peanuts in their natural shells may be fine, while the prepackaged versions fried in vegetable oils may be problematic. The coating or skin of the nut may also be a problem because of its high phytic acid content. This can cause digestive problems and also interfere with the absorption of nutrients. One recommendation to avoid this issue is prolonged soaking of the raw nuts for several hours prior to toasting them at home.

Including small amounts of nuts in our diets can bring potential health benefits. They do provide us with the good mono- and polyunsaturated fats, vitamin E, heart-healthy compounds called sterols, anti-inflammatory components, and they also pack a potent antioxidant punch. Consuming nuts at least twice a week has been associated with significant reductions in the risk of dying from coronary heart disease. The decreased risk is not small; the numbers are dramatic and run from 35 to 50 percent depending on the study population. In intervention studies where individuals are given nuts to eat over time, researchers consistently see a lowering of the bad (LDL) cholesterol. Just three ounces of pistachio nuts per day have been shown to lower the "bad" cholesterol by almost 12 percent in just one month.

The high levels of omega-3 fatty acids in walnuts have been noted by researchers, and a recent study in the journal *Nutrition & Cardiovascular Diseases* (2007) showed that when adults consumed about four walnuts per day, the blood levels of the anti-inflammatory omega-3 EPA increased by an incredible 300 percent. In cases of acne, taking EPA directly through fish oil is probably a better way to go since it takes about 1–2 grams of EPA to significantly reduce inflammation. It would take handfuls of walnuts to get to that therapeutic EPA level.

Dr. Venket Rao and his colleagues at the University of Toronto recently investigated almonds and blood sugar, and they found that almonds had very beneficial effects. Specifically, they reported in the *Journal of Nutrition* (2006) that raw, unblanched almonds prevent blood-sugar spiking, which otherwise occurs after consumption of processed carbohydrates (e.g., white bread). Almonds lowered blood glucose, prevented insulin elevations, and decreased oxidative stress. Almonds, walnuts, and pure cocoa powder are all foods once feared, and now we know that they may actually be beneficial to the human skin. All are certainly worth some experimentation.

Despite the fear that nuts are calorie-dense and consumption will cause weight gain, research has actually shown that those who moderately consume nuts on a regular basis weigh less than those who do not. Intervention studies also indicate that participants consuming nuts do not gain the expected weight due to increasing nut intake, and although much more research is needed, it appears that nuts are more satiating and may increase the use of fat as an energy source. The key is in moderation; a palm-sized or one-ounce serving of the nuts that do not aggravate you, rather than a donut, margarine-based muffin, or Danish would clearly be a better option. Walnuts are a significant source of anti-inflammatory omega-3 fatty acids, and they also contain the sleep-regulating and potent antioxidant chemical called melatonin.

PURPLE/DEEP RED FOODS

Foods that contain purple-colored pigments called anthocyanins are now being recognized as extra special when it comes to antioxidant support and maintaining blood flow to the skin. Examples of such foods include blueberries, bilberries (European blueberry), dark cherries, purple carrots (yes, they come in purple too!), pomegranates, acai, purple sweet potatoes, purple cauliflower, black grapes, and beets. The purple pigments offer significant antioxidant protection and have also been shown to exert a significant anti-inflammatory effect capable of reducing pain. Acai has become a very popular choice in North America for the promotion of healthy skin. The Brazilian berry is not only incredibly delicious, but based on new research, it has emerged as an antioxidant leader in the purple/red food category. The purple anthocyanins in acai may improve blood flow and support the collagen or the scaffolding of the skin. Booster Juice, the renowned North American juice bar chain, has made brilliant use of acai by combining it with other antioxidants in healthy smoothies. You can also find matcha green tea at your local Booster Juice location. Recently, consumption of anthocyanin-rich cherries for one month was shown to decrease the levels of the inflammatory marker C-reactive protein in adults by an impressive 25 percent. The purple sweet potato is revered as a health food in Japan, where research has shown that it improves blood flow and prevents spiking of blood sugar and insulin release. The extract of this purple spud has found its way into health drinks in Japan and North America.

GREEN FOODS

Dark green vegetables of all sorts contain magnesium, an important mineral that can help put the brakes on the inflammation cascade. Magnesium makes up an important part of the green pigment of plants called chlorophyll, so if you are looking at a green vegetable, you are looking at magnesium. Given that we fall short on daily serv-ings of fruits and vegetables, it should not be surprising that more than half of the U.S. population does not meet even the minimum recom-mendations for daily intake of magnesium. In a study published in the *Journal of the American College of Nutrition* (2005), researchers from the Medical University of South Carolina showed that in almost four thousand adults, those with low dietary magnesium intake (50 percent RDA) were about three times more likely (versus those meeting the RDA) to have levels of C-reactive protein that are in the danger zone. C-reactive protein is a well-recognized blood marker of inflammation. Doctors have recently been making connections between elevations in this inflammatory marker and the risk of chronic medical conditions. There are numerous experimental studies showing that magnesium deficiency causes an elevated production of both inflammatory chemi-cals and free radicals. It is also of note that inadequate dietary mag-nesium intake is well known to increase substance P release. Do you remember our brief discussion of substance P? It is most well-known as a nervous system chemical that promotes pain in the human body; however, recently it has also been shown to be involved in the acne process by promoting sebum production. Research has also shown that magnesium reduces an overactive stress response in individuals experiencing competitive stress. As we will discuss later, nutritional considerations in the stress-acne cycle are very important.

EGGS

Eggs have been an important source of nutrition for centuries, although modern egg production has chipped away at some of those nutritional benefits. In particular, alterations to the typical diet of poultry (i.e., feeding them strictly grains) caused a decline in the omega-3 content of mass-produced eggs. At one time, eggs were very rich in omega-3 fatty acids due to the natural diet of greens, seeds, and small insects. Nutrition expert Dr. Artemis Simopoulos made note of this in the *Journal of Nutrition* (2001) when she reported the omega-3 content of eggs from foraging hens roaming the Mediterranean coun-tryside. The typical North American mass-produced egg has a ratio of omega-6 to omega-3 of around 20:1, which very much reflects our high overall dietary intake of omega-6 fatty acids. The reason for this high omega-6 content is that most mass-produced eggs are from chickens fed a diet very high in corn and grains. The omega-3 to omega-6 ratio of the wild eggs in the Greek islands is a near perfect 1:1 match, with the added bonus of lower levels of less-desirable fats.

In the context of the Clear Skin Diet, we highlight omega-3–enriched eggs because they have been shown to be an anti-inflammatory food. In a double-blind, controlled study with forty-two healthy volunteers, researchers showed that consuming two omega-3 eggs daily (total 200 mg of EPA/DHA) dampened inflammatory markers. Writing in the journal *Nutrition, Metabolism & Cardiovascular Diseases* (2005), Dr. Hossein Fakhrzadeh and colleagues reported that after six weeks of eating the omega-3 eggs (control was standard supermarket egg), the levels of the most important marker of inflammation, C-reactive protein, dropped significantly. What's more, there was also a drop in insulin levels, indicating the omega-3 eggs may have helped balance blood sugar—as we will see, this is yet another bonus for acne improvement.

After the publication of Dr. Logan's book *The Brain Diet*, where eggs were discussed as a "brain food," he was queried about the cooking of eggs, and the question came up: Does cooking destroy the omega-3 fatty acids? Feeding hens a diet rich in vitamin E can definitely stabilize the omega-3 inside the eggs in the raw state; however, it had been speculated that cooking might destroy the omega-3. A joint investigation by researchers from Spain and Germany took up this question. They found that cooking processes have very little effect at all on the omega-3 content of the eggs. Scrambling, poaching, and overall less cooking time may offer an advantage over hard-boiling due to less overall breakdown of fats within the eggs. Therefore, the current evidence suggests that the omega-3 levels are preserved within the shells and are well capable of making a physiological difference in the body when consumed as part of a healthy diet.

Final Thoughts

In general, the fiber-containing whole grains, fruits and vegetables, and seafood are all anti-inflammatory foods that have been shown to lower the inflammatory marker CRP. In one study, cardiovascular

---

Acne Nutrient Highlight – Selenium

What is it?

Selenium is a minor mineral that pulls quite a bit of weight in the body. Selenium is required for the function of many enzymes throughout the body, including those involved in the immune and antioxidant defense systems. Sources include whole grains, nuts, seafood, salmon, and halibut.

Why is it of value?

Selenium is critical to the workings of the antioxidant system, allowing one of the most important antioxidants in the human body, glutathione, to do its job. Selenium has been shown to work synergistically with, and to preserve the levels of, other antioxidants. The selenium-dependent enzyme that controls glutathione is low in acne patients, and low levels of blood selenium have also been documented. Research showed that selenium and a small amount of vitamin E can improve acne, particularly in those with low baseline glutathione enzyme activity. At least five studies have shown that low selenium levels are associated with lowered mood states, and clinical studies show supplementation can improve symptoms of minor depression and anxiety.

---

patients were placed on a diet whereby fiber intake was increased from 14 to 32 grams per day. CRP levels were decreased by more than 40 percent during the course of two years on the fiber-rich diet. In a study published in the *Journal of Nutrition* (2004), researchers showed that among almost four thousand subjects, those with the lowest dietary fiber intake had a 50 percent higher risk of having elevated levels of CRP than those with high fiber intake. Researchers from the Medical University of South Carolina reported similar results in the *American Journal of Cardiology* (2003), where the level of CRP was significantly lower (50 percent) among those in the highest fiber group.

Research shows that the preparation of foods might also be important in lowering oxidative stress and inflammation. Cooking and processing of foods using high heat and the absence of moisture (high and dry heat) lead to the formation of chemicals called advanced glycation end products (AGEs) in food. When sugary sauces or marinades are

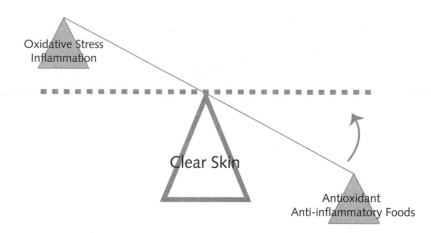

Oxidative Stress
Inflammation

Clear Skin

Antioxidant
Anti-inflammatory Foods

used on meats cooked on a dry heat, the AGE levels are very high. These dietary AGEs, when consumed by even healthy adults, increase the oxidative-stress burden and promote inflammation in humans. Researchers from Mount Sinai School of Medicine in New York recently showed that dietary restriction of high-AGE foods, and instructions on using boiling and stewing versus deep-frying and high-dry heat, leads to a dramatic reduction in AGEs circulating in the bloodstream. Perhaps most important, a low dietary AGE plan is associated with significant reductions in inflammatory chemicals at the genetic level. Just one more example of how diet can influence genes despite our genetic susceptibilities. Incorporating a low-AGE diet by avoiding high-AGE foods and utilizing boiling, stewing, poaching, and steaming is yet another way to minimize your oxidative-stress load and low-grade inflammation and reduce the flames of acne.

Chapter Key Points

✔ Inflammation is at the core of acne.
✔ Oxidative stress fans the flames of inflammation.
✔ Our innate antioxidant defense system is dependent upon dietary antioxidants.
✔ The standard American diet (SAD) promotes inflammation.
✔ Stress promotes inflammation.
✔ Oil glands produce not only sebum, they also manufacture inflammatory chemicals.

✔ Fish oil, especially EPA (1–2 grams), blocks the production of the inflammatory chemicals.

✔ Nicotinamide (vitamin B3 derivative) and zinc have anti-inflammatory properties and slow sebum production. Nicotinamide is absorbed through the skin when applied topically.

✔ Antioxidants—Vitamins A and E, lipoic acid, selenium, lycopene, and green tea all have antiacne potential. Anti-inflammatory culinary herbs such as ginger and turmeric may also play a role.

✔ Acne patients are less-frequent consumers of antioxidant, anti-inflammatory–rich fruits, vegetables, and fish.

✔ Food preparation with high heat in the absence of water (moisture) also promotes inflammation and oxidative stress.

4

Hormones and the Clear Skin Diet

Androgens

Hormones are a huge player in the development of acne, and although the precise mechanisms behind their powerful influence remain unknown, we do know that androgens gum up the follicle by stimulating sebum production. Androgens, of course, are the so-called "male" hormones manufactured by both the testes and the adrenal glands, and they are responsible for sexual development and secondary sex characteristics. The most well-known androgens are testosterone and its breakdown product, dihydrotestosterone. Women also manufacture androgens, albeit in smaller amounts via the ovaries and the adrenal glands, which help to maintain bone density and sexual desire. One of the long-recognized side effects of administering androgen compounds, anabolic steroids, and testosterone is the development of acne.

How can we be so sure that androgens are involved in the acne process? Well, for starters, there are rare circumstances in which certain individuals are completely insensitive to androgens and lack receptors for androgens to bind to—these folks do not produce sebum, and they never develop acne. In contrast, when certain cancers of the ovary or adrenal glands cause excessive secretion of androgens, the disease may come to light because it is accompanied by acne. In some cases, the severity of acne is also associated with higher levels of blood androgens and the administration of testosterone, and the chief precursor to testosterone, called DHEA (dehydroepiandrosterone, made by the adrenal glands), causes growth and increased productivity of the sebaceous glands. The levels of DHEA can start rising well before puberty, when the adrenal glands start producing this chemical. This is the time when acne begins to show up in genetically susceptible pre-teens.

The androgens circulate around the body and then latch onto receptors at various sites. We now know that there are androgen receptors in the basement of the sebaceous glands (sebum-producing glands) and also in cells that line the follicle canal. Testosterone and dihydrotestosterone (DHT) are more than capable of binding onto these receptors within the pilosebaceous unit. DHT may be the real culprit because it binds onto androgen receptors much more efficiently and is said to be five to ten times more powerful than testosterone when it comes to the stimulating the hormonally influenced glands. Testosterone is converted into DHT by an enzyme called 5-alpha-reductase (5αR) (now stay with us—we don't want to lose you at 5αR; it's not as complicated as you might think), and it has been shown that the activity of 5αR is greater in the sebaceous glands of acne-prone skin. Greater activity of 5αR means more DHT available in acne-prone skin, which means even more sebum to gum up your follicles and more food for bacteria/yeasts, with the net result of more inflammation. The conversion of DHEA into testosterone also requires the work of a couple of enzymes, and these, too, are at work in the human skin. DHEA from the adrenal glands is first converted into androstenedione through the work of 3β-HSD (3-beta-hydroxysteroid dehydrogenase), and then androstenedione is converted into testosterone by 17β-HSD (17-beta-hydroxysteroid dehydrogenase).

I'm sure by now you are wondering why we are giving you a tutorial on these conversion enzymes with their long chemical names, and you probably want to know what it all means from a practical standpoint. Well, there is a growing body of research that demonstrates that diet can influence the activity of these enzymes and overall levels of these hormones. Much of what we know about this area has evolved from studies related to hormonally influenced cancers such as those of the breast and prostate. Accumulating evidence has linked higher circulating androgens with increased risk of both breast and prostate cancers, while a host of epidemiological studies have shown that regional

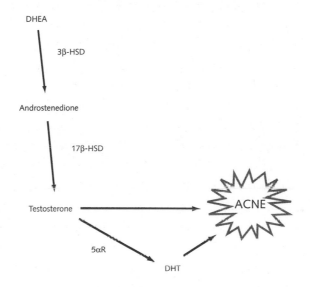

dietary differences might play a role in the development of both of these hormonal cancers. Dr. Danby points out that the very same group of enzymes in the pilosebaceous unit are also likely responsible for converting the four (or more) hormones in milk into DHT. Even more importantly, two of these hormones are already "5αR reduced" in the cow mammary gland. In simple terms, this means that the hormones are already biologically converted into active form and go straight to the androgen receptor regardless of location—sebaceous gland, follicular canal, breast tissue, or prostate tissue. The research that has uncovered nutritional elements that are potentially breast and prostate cancer protective is relevant to acne patients. We say this because research in the *European Journal of Cancer Prevention* (1996) shows that acne in the teen years is associated with an increased risk of later breast cancer, and a study in the *American Journal of Epidemiology* (2005) shows that teen boys with acne are more likely to go on to have prostate cancer later in life. Long-term dietary changes may help with acne today, and also positively influence the risk of hormonal cancers years later.

Of course, like many medical conditions, there is a family history connection to breast and prostate cancer, so those who try to negate dietary influences use the old acne excuse that it's all about genetics. There is a problem with that old argument, though, because research has shown that despite the much lower rates of prostate cancer among older Japanese men, the risk becomes much higher in Western nations, and in second- and third-generation Japanese-American men, the risk is the same as in Caucasians. The same environmental influences are at play in considering the risk of breast cancer among Japanese women. The rates of breast cancer through the 1980s were up to six times lower in Japan, and yet when Japanese women migrate to Western countries the rates are much closer to those of Caucasian women. While discussions on the low rates of breast and prostate cancer in Japan compared to North America are plastered all over the Internet, it is important to point out that the gap between the rates in Japan and in Western countries is rapidly being narrowed. The rates of breast and prostate cancers in Japan have seen dramatic increases in recent years, a rise that coincides with the Westernization of the traditional Japanese diet. It is just way too easy to write off differences in the rates of diseases, including acne, with the genetics card. What is more likely is that environment, including diet and stressors, influences genetic mechanisms in hormonally influenced conditions. This is the emerging science of nutrigenomics at work.

While certain dietary items like soy have been extolled as magic foods that prevent breast and prostate cancers, it is the totality of the Japanese diet that makes it protective. Collectively, it is the moderate intake of soy, fish and seafood, green tea, seaweed, a plentiful variety of fruits and vegetables, less sugar, less animal fat, less trans fats, less vegetable oils, more fiber, more antioxidants, more omega-3 fatty acids, and less sugars and processed foods that would otherwise spike insulin levels—these are the antiacne features of the traditional Japanese diet, the features that resulted in rates of acne that were half that of American teens just forty short years ago. Many of the dietary items that are part of the traditional Japanese diet have been shown to influence androgens and other hormones in humans. However, the most profound influence that kept the incidence of cancers and acne low in Japan may have been the *absence* of the Western diet.

We have previously discussed the critically important omega-3 fatty acids and their potential application in acne. In addition to suppressing the inflammatory pathways that are active in acne, these oils may also be influencing the hormonal aspects of acne. Researchers have found that testosterone actually lowers the blood levels of one key omega-3 fatty acid. Reporting in the *American Journal of Clinical Nutrition* (2004), researchers from the Netherlands discovered that female hormones (which are, generally speaking, protective of acne) promote higher concentrations of omega-3 DHA—not just by a little bit—the increase was 42 percent. Amazingly, when testosterone was administered to the healthy adults, there was a 22 percent decrease in blood DHA levels. Since DHA has anti-inflammatory properties and can be retro-converted back into the anti-inflammatory omega-3 EPA, these results have important hormonal-acne implications.

Excess dietary fat, and saturated fat in particular, has been shown in a large number of studies to influence blood levels of androgens. One of the first human studies to document a diet-hormone connection was in 1984 by Dr. Esa Hamalainen and colleagues from the University of Helsinki in Finland. This team showed that by switching from a diet high in saturated animal fat to one with 38 percent less fat and more inclusive of healthier polyunsaturated fats for six weeks, significant reductions resulted in androstenedione and testosterone in the blood. So it seems that these "good" fats have a special relationship with testosterone—higher testosterone may lower important omega-3 fatty acid levels, while administration of the oils might also lower testosterone.

Over the years, separate international groups have found similar relationships between saturated fat and increased androgens in adults. Writing in the journal *Nutrition and Cancer* (2000), researchers from Japan found that a higher intake of the EPA and DHA omega-3 fatty acids found in fish oil was associated with lower circulating testosterone. Recently the same group, led by Dr. Chisato Nagata of Gifu University, reported that higher total dietary fat (and saturated fat in particular) is associated with higher blood DHEA levels.

Studies where benefits are described from a "low-fat diet" might be due to a number of reasons related to the fat. Was the diet beneficial due to a reduction in saturated animal fat, trans/hydrogenated oils, or the omega-6 excesses of vegetable oils? We also wonder if saturated fat itself is a problem or if the problem comes from the types of fat the animal is fed during rearing. A corn/grain-based diet is standard fare for most livestock, and it results in a very high omega-6 content and higher overall fat in meat compared to roaming animals that feed on grasses—the meat from these free-range animals has less fat overall and a much higher level of omega-3 fats.

In 2001, Italian researchers placed more than fifty healthy women (in the highest testosterone bracket for age) on a controlled diet rich in whole grains, vegetables, omega-3 fatty acids, monounsaturated fat (olive oil), soy-foods, and fiber, but low in animal fat and any processed foods that spike blood sugar. An additional fifty-two women acted as controls by consuming a typical Western diet. After four and a half months, those consuming the low-fat, high-fiber diet had increased levels of sex-hormone-binding globulin (this binding protein has a firm grip on otherwise free and active androgens in circulation) and decreased levels of total blood testosterone. We will discuss the naturally occurring hormonal binding proteins in more detail later.

Fiber is an important dietary component when it comes to androgens. As long ago as 1979, it was reported that switching from a traditional high-fiber diet to one much lower in fiber can cause an increase in urinary androgen levels. In a study published in the journal *Cancer* (1994), researchers from Tufts University showed that when a typical high-fat, low-fiber Western diet was switched to one with about

Daily Fiber Requirements

Age	Daily Fiber* Needed
Men 14–50	38 g
Women 14–50	25 g
Men over 50	30 g
Women over 50	21 g
Children 2–13	5 g

*The recommended daily Adequate Intake (AI) of total fiber as per the U.S. National Academy of Sciences and Health Canada. Note that the typical fiber intake for adults is currently 13 grams.

half the fat and more than three times the fiber, there were significant decreases in blood levels of testosterone and androstenedione among forty-eight healthy females. Following this, researchers from the National Cancer Institute looked at dietary fat and fiber for ten weeks in healthy males—they showed that a similar low-fat, high-fiber diet led to lower total testosterone levels, including a 13 percent decrease in circulating testosterone and urinary testosterone excretion versus the high-fat, low-fiber diet.

More recently, Dr. Christina Wang and colleagues from UCLA Medical Center reported on the influence of an eight-week dietary intervention on androgens in middle-aged males. Writing in the *Journal of Clinical Endocrinology and Metabolism* (2005), they reported that after the low-fat, high-fiber diet there were significant decreases in blood testosterone, androstenedione, DHT, and DHEA. The total effects of the dietary change were similar to previous reports and amounted to a 12 percent decrease in circulating androgens. The amount of dietary fiber consumed each day through the eight weeks was typical of the amount consumed in traditional diets uninfluenced by the processing and sugars of the modern Western diet. We are about 33 percent lower on the fiber scale compared to what was consumed in traditional diets just a century ago. Depending on age and gender, North Americans are, on the average, 7 to 25 grams short of optimal daily fiber intake.

A separate area of investigation concerning diet and hormones revolves around soy food consumption. As mentioned, the preponderance of the evidence suggests that it is the totality of the healthy, traditional Japanese diet that protects against breast and prostate cancers—however, it is worth examining the soy research just to highlight how it can make a difference. In a study published in *Nutrition and Cancer* (2000), it was once again Dr. Chisato Nagata of Gifu University in Japan at work, this time showing that greater soy product consumption was associated with lower levels of free and bound testosterone in the blood of Japanese men. This was an interesting finding because experimental studies have shown that the naturally occurring plant flavonoids called isoflavones (plant estrogens) are capable of inhibiting the androgen-forming and acne-promoting enzymes 17β-HSD and 5αR. Fermented soy products such as miso, natto, and tempeh appear to provide isoflavones that are more bio-available, or better absorbed for use in the body. Dr. Nagata's group found that it was specifically the greater isoflavone consumption that was related to lower levels of blood androgens. They found a typical intake of isoflavones to be around 22 mg per day, right in line with the larger research of Dr. Yumiko Nakamura from Japan's National Institute of Health Sciences, who found that national consumption of isoflavones is around 28 mg per day. The North American intake of isoflavones is around only 5 mg per day.

In a study in the *British Journal of Nutrition* (2000), researchers from Australia switched the protein source of healthy adult males from meat to tofu (calories remained the same) for one month. The meat diet resulted in greater concentrations of testosterone relative to estrogens, while the tofu diet resulted in less freely available testosterone in circulation. Researchers from the hospital where Dr. Logan was born, the Royal Victoria Hospital in Belfast, Northern Ireland, showed that baked goods made with soy flour can influence androgen levels. Reporting in the *European Journal of Clinical Nutrition* (2003), they discovered that when healthy males ate three soy-flour-based scones (versus wheat-flour scones) every day for six weeks, there were significant effects on circulating testosterone. Total blood testosterone was decreased in those consuming the soy scones, and there was also a decrease in blood markers of oxidative stress. The latter finding was not surprising because a number of studies have shown that, like most flavonoids, isoflavones have strong antioxidant activity. The daily consumption of isoflavones was about four times that of the typical Japanese diet. We should point out that isoflavone-rich foods such as miso, tofu, soy milk, and tempeh are not to be confused with dietary supplements containing isoflavones that have been isolated out of the whole food and encapsulated. There is more unknown than known about these high-dose supplements of isolated isoflavones—they may carry health risks by disturbing the natural hormonal interactions of the body over time.

The typical Western diet is also an acid-heavy diet due to the over-consumption of meat-based proteins and processed grains. Fruits and vegetables, on the other hand, are very alkaline and capable of neutralizing the acids formed by meats and grains in the body. The impact of a diet top-heavy in meats and processed grains has been the subject of much scientific inquiry and discussion by lay websites. The reason is because an acidic diet consumed on a regular basis over many years, in the absence of alkaline fruits and vegetables, can promote osteoporosis. When a typical Western diet is consumed, calcium is leached out of the bones in an effort to neutralize acids formed by too many grains and meat-based protein. The acidic meal resulting in osteoporosis obviously doesn't happen overnight—one meal won't make or break osteoporosis; the problem occurs when acid meals are strung together and consumed on a regular basis. There are acne-hormonal consequences to this acid-heavy diet devoid of fruits and vegetables. Researchers investigating the Western diet–osteoporosis connection placed a group of healthy volunteers on a typical acid-forming diet and found that there were fairly rapid elevations in the stress hormone cortisol. The results, published in the *American Journal of Physiology and Renal Physiology* (2003), also showed that neutralizing the otherwise acid-heavy Western diet reduced the secretion of cortisol in these adults. Since cortisol is known to be elevated in acne patients, and it in turn may be influencing other inflammatory chemicals, the need for an alkaline diet rich in fruits and vegetables may be even more critical.

There are lots of other healthy foods that may influence the enzymes that ultimately control the "strength" of androgens. Certain components of the flavonoid-rich family of foods can dampen down the activity of those hormonal enzymes 3β-HSD, 17β-HSD and 5αR. For example, quercetin is a flavonoid found in high amounts in berries, dark grapes, red wine, kale, broccoli, tomatoes, apples, green beans, honey, and peppers. Quercetin has been shown to inhibit 3β-HSD and 17β-HSD more effectively than many other flavonoids under experimental circumstances. Naturally occurring chemicals called flavanones, such as naringenin in citrus fruits; coumestans in bean shoots, alfalfa, spinach, and sunflower seeds; as well as lignans found in cereals, flaxseeds, and fruits and vegetables, can all make a contribution to inhibiting the 17β-HSD androgen-converting enzyme.

Green tea contains the important antioxidant chemical called EGCG, which, along with the omega-3 fatty acid EPA and gamma-linolenic acid (GLA, from evening primrose and borage oils), have all been shown to inhibit the activity of 5αR. Dr. Shutsung Liao of the University of Chicago was the first to report, in 1992, that GLA and EGCG reduce sebum when applied topically to the skin. In addition to directly inhibiting 5αR, there may also be other mechanisms of decreasing sebum formation. The anti-inflammatory properties of all three of these compounds, EGCG, EPA, and GLA, may play a role in the inhibition of 5αR because, as we discussed previously, researchers from the University of California (Davis) showed that turning down the inflammatory dial via inhibition of LTB4 resulted in decreased conversion of testosterone into DHT. Remember, DHT is bad news for sebum production at the bottom of the pilosebaceous unit. Remember also that EPA from fish oil and GLA from borage (and primrose oil) can diminish LTB4 production, and, therefore, since blocking LTB4 decreases DHT formation, these healthy fats can influence the final formation of DHT from testosterone.

The potential benefits of EGCG in modulating the hormonal

Considering a Bottle of Green Tea?

We are amazed at the marketing of ready-made commercial green tea drinks—convenience stores and vending machines from coast to coast promise major antioxidant support from bottled green tea beverages. We urge you to think twice about these sugary or artificially sweetened beverages. The latest USDA studies show that a cup of brewed green tea contains twenty times more of the important antioxidant and potentially acne protective EGCG than bottled ready-to-drink green teas. A 2005 study from Oregon State University found an even greater disparity—Dr. Rod Dashwood and colleagues found that freshly brewed green tea had up to one hundred times more antioxidants than these bottled teas.

Consider that one of these large green tea bottles in the fridge of your local store has more than forty-two grams of sugar and 175 calories! This is not an antiacne beverage. In the Oregon State press release on bottled green tea, Dr. Dashwood stated: "Many of the currently available cold bottled teas sold in the United States are more like diluted sugar water than something that may help protect your health."

aspects of acne did not escape all dermatologists; Dr. James Shaw of the University of Toronto was aware of the green tea research and made note of the potential value of EGCG in acne treatment. Writing in the *Archives of Dermatology* (2001), he referenced the $5\alpha R$ inhibiting properties of EGCG and suggested there may be potential. Six years later we are still awaiting further exploration of green tea and its EGCG component in the treatment of acne.

In addition to the possible hormonal influences of green tea on acne, there are other mechanisms whereby green tea can affect the acne process. As previously mentioned, green tea is a potent anti-inflammatory beverage rich in naturally occurring antioxidant cat-

---

Matcha

The highest grade of green tea is Japanese matcha—a fine powder of green tea leaves. Matcha green tea is grown under specific conditions, including the avoidance of direct sunlight on the leaves. In 2003, researchers from the University of Colorado found that the concentration of EGCG available from drinking matcha is up to 137 times greater than the amount of EGCG available from other commercially available green teas. Matcha is also a perfect addition to baked goods, yogurts, and smoothies. Mix with hot Rice Dream or soy milk for a hot matcha latte.

Packaged matcha green tea from Japan is available at all North American Booster Juice locations and a www.kenkonutrition.com.

---

echins. There is yet another important aspect of green tea that makes it a worthwhile choice in cases of acne—research in the *Annals of Nutrition & Metabolism* (2005) shows that it can *increase* blood levels of both zinc and selenium. As we are sure you recall, both zinc and selenium are critical nutrients in the body's fight against the development and progression of acne. Green tea also has some antistress properties, which we will take up in chapter 6, "The Brain-Skin Connection."

Astaxanthin is a naturally occurring carotenoid chemical that gives fish and seafood a pinkish-red color. A number of recent studies have focused in on astaxanthin, with data showing that it has up to five

Detox for Acne?

The concept of "detoxification" for acne still gets thrown around in various resources, including the Internet. Life-changing dietary detox plans abound, and today the term "detox" is so vague that it has become difficult to define. The plans can range from extreme fasting, to juice only, and yet others involve the temporary use of expensive supplements, often with harsh chemicals. We caution against such approaches. The human body is equipped with a very proficient detoxification system, one that is entirely reliant upon a variety of important nutrients—not the lack of nutrients via fasting, or lack of protein via juicing.

Your ability to detoxify through the liver and gastrointestinal tract, the main organs of detox, is only as good as the quality of your diet. Intake of dietary fiber, maintenance of friendly bacteria in the GI tract, and providing nutrients that support the liver in the handling of toxins are the cornerstones to efficient elimination. The detox issue in acne relates to the disposition of hormones—if the acne-promoting hormones are not eliminated efficiently, they can be recirculated in the active form.

Researchers from Japan reported in the *Tohoku Journal of Experimental Medicine* (1956) that nutritional support of liver detoxification can improve acne. Specifically they showed that administration of glucuronic acid (a nutrient that helps transform and eliminate sex hormones) in the liver successfully improved acne in 78 percent of cases. Since then an abundance of research has shown that support of liver detox and the handling of sex hormones is enhanced via *Brassica* family vegetables (e.g., kale, broccoli, Brussels sprouts). Onions, garlic, leeks, green tea, turmeric, pomegranates, ginger, honey, and citrus components can also help with normal hormonal detoxification. Research data is lacking in acne; however, the take-home message is that the "ultimate detox diet" reflects what has been long-promoted for chronic disease and general health—one with a colorful variety of plants and quality, lean-protein sources.

hundred times the antioxidant capacity of vitamin E and ten times the antioxidant capacity of beta-carotene. This in itself would make it advantageous in acne; however, another recent study in the *Journal of Herbal Pharmacotherapy* (2005) shows that it can also inhibit 5αR. Salmon, rich in both omega-3 fatty acids and astaxanthin, emerges as a core dietary choice in the Clear Skin Diet plan.

Insulin-Like Growth Factor

Outside the androgens, there are other hormonal influences on acne. One hormone now known to be involved in the acne process is insulin-like growth factor-1 (IGF-1). IGF-1 is structurally similar to the blood-sugar-regulating hormone insulin, although the two hormones work in different ways. IGF-1 is an anabolic hormone directly involved in growth and development, particularly through the growth spurt at puberty when levels of IGF-1 are typically much higher. Blood levels of IGF-1 are much lower before puberty and in old age. In 1995, researchers from the Jikei University School of Medicine in

---

Acne Nutrient Highlight—Epigallocatechin-3-Gallate (EGCG)

What is it?

EGCG is a phytochemical in the polyphenol family. The research on this key antioxidant continues to build in the cardiovascular, cancer, diabetes, neurodegenerative, and obesity arenas. EGCG occurs in tea, although it is highest in Japanese matcha green tea. Substantial amounts can be found in loose Japanese tea, followed by lesser amounts in white tea, oolong tea, and traditional English-style black tea.

Why is it of value?

The EGCG polyphenol from green tea has been suggested to be helpful in acne through its well-documented anti-inflammatory and antioxidant activity. Recently it has also been reported that since it is known to possess 5-α-reductase (5αR) inhibiting properties, EGCG may also influence hormonal aspects of acne. Since 5αR is responsible for production of the acne-promoting hormone dihydrotestosterone, slowing down this process may be of benefit.

Japan put IGF-1 on the acne map when they showed that the levels of IGF-1 in 82 acne patients were higher than age-matched controls without acne. On the other hand, human studies show that injections of synthetic IGF-1 lead to elevations in testosterone, androstenedione, and, yes, you guessed it—acne.

Things move very slowly in acne research, and it wasn't until another decade after the Japanese study that the IGF-1 connection received proper attention. Then, in 2005, a study was published in the *Archives of Dermatology* that showed the expected associations among DHEA and DHT and acne—however, they also noted that the effect of androgens on the appearance of facial acne was dependent upon IGF-1. It seemed that IGF-1 was a bigger player than ever imagined in the development of acne in both men and women, and since the sebaceous glands have receptors for IGF-1, it was suspected that elevated levels of the hormone are probably influencing acne via stimulating the growth of the oil-producing gland.

In a follow-up study published in the *Journal of Investigative Dermatology* (2006), researchers from Penn State University showed that IGF-1 does indeed stimulate the production of fat by the cells of the sebaceous glands. They also found that insulin itself, our blood-sugar-regulating hormone, can do the same thing. This is just one more reason to suspect that the Western diet, with its bountiful variety of insulin-spiking, processed, high-sugar foods, is involved in plugging up the follicle.

More on the insulin connection in a moment, but first let's examine how diet can influence IGF-1. Once again, much of what we know about dietary influences on IGF-1 has come from investigations related to the risk of breast and prostate cancers. Elevated IGF-1 levels have been closely associated with these hormonal cancers, while in contrast, higher levels of the IGF-binding proteins are associated with a decreased risk. Remember we mentioned the sex-hormone-binding protein and how it holds on tightly to testosterone, lowering its activity levels? The same is basically true of IGF-binding proteins (BPs), except in this case they hold on to IGF-1 like a vise grip in the blood. In simple terms, if levels of these BPs dip down, that translates into more "free" IGF-1 circulating around and stimulating sebaceous glands to cause acne.

While many animal studies have shown that dietary quality can influence IGF-1, it was only in 1999 that the first human study suggested a link. Harvard researchers showed that blood levels of IGF-1 in adults are associated with red meat, and overall fat and saturated fat appeared to be a main culprit because the higher the levels of saturated fat, the lower the levels of IGF BPs. Separate groups of researchers, from the United Kingdom and Japan, have since followed up on this work and found the same relationship between increased circulating IGF-1 and saturated fat.

Researchers from Oxford, United Kingdom, were more specific with the study populations, and they showed that blood IGF-1 was 9 percent lower in 233 vegans than in 226 meat eaters. You might be thinking, *Big deal—what on earth does a 9 percent difference mean?* Actually, it means a lot, because a group of Harvard researchers previously showed in a large study that men who subsequently develop prostate cancer had an 8 percent higher IGF-1 level than those who did not go on to have prostate cancer.

This is an important point to consider; because we are examining and highlighting dietary choices that can significantly influence hormone levels, it is important to recognize that we are not talking about some form of nutritional castration. The changes in androgen levels due to diet are indeed statistically significant; however, they are not huge and are likely just enough to make a clinical difference when combined with other antiacne properties. When we look at nutritional influences on the genetics of human health, we are now beginning to understand that small changes to hormonal and other markers can have enormous benefit, particularly when considering the constellation of dietary influences as we are doing in *The Clear Skin Diet*.

Researchers from UCLA reported dramatic dietary influences on IGF-1 and IGF-binding proteins after an eleven-day diet intervention. The diet was low in fat, high in fiber, and rich in fruits, vegetables, and whole grains. The participants were overweight but otherwise healthy, and they were also asked to engage in sixty minutes of aerobic physical activity every day. After less than two weeks there was a 20 percent decrease in blood levels of IGF-1, and a 53 percent increase in IGF BPs. For participants who went further and followed the diet-and-exercise plan over the long term, there was a 55 percent reduction in IGF-1, and the IGF BPs were 150 percent higher compared to baseline. The study, published in *Cancer Causes and Control* (2002), also showed that the regimen decreased blood-insulin levels by 25 percent after just eleven days. Following this were more diet and IGF-1 studies that solidified the connection.

Researchers from Italy also showed that a change in dietary habits for five months can change IGF-1. In this case about fifty women were assigned to a group consuming a low-fat, high-fiber diet rich in omega-3 fatty acids and soy foods. There was also a reduction in both omega-6 and total saturated fats. The diet was a huge success—significant elevations in IGF BPs, decreased androgens, decreased markers of inflammation (C-reactive protein), and decreased blood sugar and insulin levels.

The relationship between milk consumption and elevated IGF-1 has been given considerable attention. Quite a few studies have shown that milk consumption is perhaps king among foods and beverages associated with higher levels of blood IGF-1. Just how great is the influence of milk on IGF-1? In a study published in the *Journal of the American Dietetic Association* (1999), researchers found that drinking three (eight-ounce) servings of nonfat or 1 percent milk for twelve weeks led to a 10 percent increase in IGF-1 blood levels among healthy men and women. Bovine, or cow-milk-derived, IGF-1 is identical to human IGF-1, and there is evidence that it can escape digestive breakdown, pass through the intestinal wall, and go to work throughout the body as an intact hormone. This may explain, at least partially, the increase in IGF-1 seen in milk drinkers. Given what we know about IGF-1 stimulating the production of oil at the sebaceous gland, is it any wonder that Harvard researchers have twice shown relationships between milk and acne?

When it comes to IGF-1, research is showing that tomatoes are quite the opposite of milk and actually may limit IGF-1 production. Researchers from the University of Bristol in the United Kingdom reported in 2003 that a diet rich in vegetables was associated with lower IGF-1 levels in 344 healthy males. Among the vegetables they found that tomatoes in particular were highly associated with low IGF-1 levels. This is interesting because it confirmed what Harvard researchers had reported two years earlier—cooked tomatoes were specifically associated with an average 32 percent less IGF-1 for each incremental serving per day. Since the absorption of the important antioxidant lycopene within tomatoes is enhanced by cooking, it could very well be the lycopene that is at work lowering IGF-1 levels. Animal studies indicate that tomato powder and lycopene added to the laboratory chow can significantly reduce blood levels of testosterone—even studies as short as four days have revealed statistical changes. This lycopene research also provides a reason why Dr. Logan has sworn for years that regular consumption of tomato juice and V8 was promoting clear skin and helping keep his acne at bay—something sensed long before we knew there were 14 milligrams of lycopene in a tiny 5.5-ounce can of Campbell's tomato juice, and long before there was knowledge about IGF-1 and acne.

In addition to diet, IGF-1 may be influenced by other factors including psychological stress and environmental pollutants. We will discuss the relationship between stress and acne in depth later, although the connection between IGF-1 and pollutants warrants mention. Italian researchers writing in the *International Journal of Environmental Health* (2004) reported that working outdoors (close to traffic), in a typical urban environment with significant exposure to air pollutants such as benzenes, may lead to significant elevations in blood IGF-1 levels. This might provide yet another reason why the rates of adult acne are on the rise in our world filled with environmental toxins. Some research, including a study in the *Indian Journal of Dermatology, Venereology and Leprology* (1980), has shown that overall rates of acne are higher in urban environments relative to rural areas. The reason could be greater adherence to more traditional diets in rural environments, the reduction in air pollutants relative to the city, lower levels of stress, or, most likely, a combination of all factors in a genetically susceptible individual.

Insulin

When Dr. Loren Cordain's team showed that acne is pretty much nonexistent among the Kitavan Islanders of Papua New Guinea and the Aché community of Paraguay, it was the low-glycemic load of the two traditional diets that jumped off the page. The glycemic load is an extension of the concept of the glycemic index (GI) of foods, a standard research reference that provides a guide to how rapidly 50 grams of a particular carbohydrate turns into blood sugar. The problem with GI is that it doesn't provide information on how much of that carbohydrate is in a *serving* of a particular food. This determination of the carbohydrate content per serving is termed "glycemic load." Perhaps the best example to show the shortcomings of the GI is in comparing a carrot to a white potato—both have a very high GI, and many people were avoiding carrots because of the high GI and the impression that they spike blood sugar. However, carrots have a very low carbohydrate content, so you would have to eat four and a half cups of cooked carrots to match the blood-sugar-spiking potential of just one baked potato because the glycemic load of carrots is much smaller. There are mathematical equations used to determine glycemic load from glycemic index, but there is no reason to make this story more complex—in practical terms, just remember that glycemic load takes into account the amount of carbohydrate in particular foods and it still represents the ability of foods to spike blood sugar. The overall dietary glycemic load is the sum of the glycemic loads for all foods consumed in the diet, and a low dietary glycemic load (GL) is characteristic of the antiacne diets of the Kitavans, the Aché, and virtually all traditional diets. In contrast, about half the daily calories consumed in the typical Western diet are from processed sugars, processed grains, white potatoes and dairy items known to be highly glycemic and therefore well capable of spiking blood sugar.

Meals that are high-glycemic (high GI or GL) cause rapid elevations of insulin that can remain high for hours after consumption. Insulin rushes out into the blood after meals, beverages, and snacks to assist in getting sugar into our cells for energy and maintenance of normal functions. Insulin levels rise particularly high when blood sugar spikes rapidly, and over time the chronic consumption of high-glycemic meals and snacks leads to chronically elevated blood-insulin levels. An individual who makes a long-term habit of choosing high-glycemic foods and drinks runs a very high risk of developing what is called insulin resistance. This means the receptors that normally bind insulin are no longer responding well to normal levels of insulin. The cell has a hearing problem when insulin knocks at the cellular door.

The body tries to knock louder by having the pancreas pump out more insulin. This sets the stage for a host of chronic medical conditions including type 2 diabetes and cardiovascular disease. The connection between spiking blood sugar, chronically elevated insulin, and diabetes is well established, but you might be wondering, How does it relate to acne?

For years there have been hints of problems with blood sugar and insulin in acne. Japanese researchers reported in the *Tohoku Journal of Experimental Medicine* (1956) that half their acne patients showed problems with the sugar loads of glucose-tolerance tests. They focused their attention on how sugar levels fluctuate in the skin following sugar ingestion. After a glucose tolerance test, the skin sugar levels should drop back to baseline in approximately sixty minutes—in patients with acne, the time to recover to baseline levels was 226 minutes. Clearly the glucose levels in the skin were remaining high for extended periods. Two years later, in a study published in the *Canadian Medical Association Journal* (1958), acne was described as "diabetes of the skin." Modern research is now backing up this fifty-year-old view; however, before we discuss the more recent advances, let's return to the historical research avenues.

Researchers from the United Kingdom reported in the *British Journal of Dermatology* (1963) that patients with acne dump significantly more glucose into the urine, and that a higher urinary level of glucose is associated with the severity of acne. We also have a sprinkling of small international studies from the late 50s and 60s that show the classic type 2 diabetes medicine tolbutamide is effective in the treatment of acne. Researchers from the University of Minnesota reported in the journal of the *New York Academy of Sciences* (1968) that a now discontinued antdiabetic drug, phenformin, was also effective in treating acne. No one could really explain it—Canadian researchers had found that the metabolism of glucose within the skin of acne patients was impaired, but it still didn't explain the role of blood sugar and insulin in the acne process.

Like many novel areas of acne research, the preliminary studies using insulin-modulating drugs were never followed up, and there wasn't another mention of it for almost forty years. At the dawn of the new millennium, it was reported that newer drug classes used to treat type 2 diabetes are helpful in alleviating acne in adult women with polycystic ovary syndrome (PCO). Patients with PCO have been well documented to have elevated blood levels of free androgens, insulin, IGF-1, and, as you might imagine with this trio of hormonal players, they are also more prone to acne. As witnessed in women with PCO and/or excess abdominal fat, we now know that chronically elevated blood-insulin levels can stimulate androgen production from the ovaries. Elevated insulin levels also suppress the production of sex-hormone-binding globulin, that little blood protein that normally holds on to and takes away the major activity of androgens.

With all of this as background, researchers from the Department of Food Science at the Royal Melbourne Institute of Technology (RMIT) set out in January 2004 to see if a high-protein (25 percent of calories), low-glycemic diet might influence acne. It was set up like a boot camp with the participants living in a nutritionally controlled environment—the research equivalent of the popular television show *Big Brother*. During the dietary boot camp, the teenagers were split into two groups, one of which was fed a diet of low-glycemic-index (GI) carbohydrates and protein-rich foods including gourmet fish, beef, and lamb, and a range of vegetables, fruits, nuts, and legumes. The control-group participants were fed a typical Western diet, high in glycemic carbohydrates including processed foods, white bread, potatoes, rice, and snack foods such as chips, cookies, and baked products. The results, published in the *Asia Pacific Journal of Clinical Nutrition* (2005), showed that the high-protein, low-glycemic diet significantly reduced circulating androgens and increased the IGF-1 binding proteins. There were clinical benefits noted as well, with the high-protein, low-glycemic diet leading to a significantly greater reduction in both total acne lesions and specific inflammatory lesions. This certainly lends credibility to Dr. Cordain's argument concerning the traditional diets of the Kitavans and the Aché—low-glycemic foods can make a difference. The research of the Australian group has now been formally published in the *Journal of the American Academy of Dermatology* (2007), and a separate diet-acne paper is reported to be in press with the *American Journal of Clinical Nutrition*.

This low-glycemic-load approach may be particularly important for teens because they actually go through a period of insulin resistance as part of the normal growth spurt during adolescence. Unsurprisingly, growth hormone rises during this time in order to stimulate the development and rapid growth that characterize the teen years. IGF-1 appears to be the main agent through which growth hormone works. One might speculate that the insulin-like action of high-circulating IGF-1 levels could put teens in a low state of blood sugar (because it is assisting the removal of sugar from the blood) unless they develop at least some resistance to this action. This documented insulin resistance of adolescence reverses back to normal when teens approach adulthood.

The precise mechanism behind insulin-spiking foods causing acne remains a mystery, although the influence of insulin on other androgens and IGF-1 likely plays a major role. It is of note that chronically elevated blood-insulin levels can promote IGF-1 and decrease the IGF-1 binding proteins. It is also of note that milk has been shown to

---

Acne Nutrient Highlight—Chromium

What is it?

Chromium is an essential mineral that has a number of functions in the human body, most notably in glucose regulation. In simple terms, chromium supports insulin in doing its job more efficiently and ultimately helps out in getting glucose from the bloodstream and into cells in an efficient manner. Chromium is also involved in fat metabolism. Sources of chromium include broccoli, grapes, oranges, grains, apples, green beans, and wheat germ.

Why is it of value?

Chromium has been shown to prevent the blood-sugar-spiking characteristic of type 2 diabetes. Epidemiological studies suggest that traditional diets that prevent spiking of blood sugar are protective against acne, and some early work with diabetes medicines in nondiabetic acne patients shows value. Medications that control blood sugar showed great promise for acne, or, as some called it, "diabetes of the skin." A preliminary study from the 1980s showed that 400 mcg of chromium improves acne. Four studies have shown that chromium supplementation can improve the symptoms of depression—including mood itself and carbohydrate cravings associated with lowered mood.

elevate not only IGF-1, but also insulin itself. As evidenced in a recent study in the *European Journal of Clinical Nutrition* (2005), the ability of milk to boost insulin levels is not a small measure. In this case, choosing milk as the daily source of protein for just seven days caused blood-insulin levels to double, even though the blood was drawn after an overnight fast! There were also signs of insulin resistance after one week. This means that the effect of milk drinking on boosting insulin levels is both significant and beyond short-term. If you combine this research with the new Penn State University work showing that both insulin and IGF-1 can stimulate the cells of the oil-producing sebaceous gland, the mechanism behind insulin-spiking foods and milk gumming up the follicles and contributing to the acne process is provided. It is even more compelling when you consider that the influence of insulin in stimulating the oil-producing cells (sebocytes) is dose-dependent, so the more you spike insulin and the longer you keep it high, the more likely you are to produce the "plugged pore" that contributes to acne.

It is worthwhile noting that one particular dietary spice, cinnamon, is gaining ground when it comes to stabilizing insulin and keeping blood sugar in check. There are lots of animal studies indicating benefit, and two preliminary studies in humans also highlight the value of cinnamon in diabetes. The studies, published in the journals *Diabetes Care* (2003) and the *European Journal of Clinical Investigation* (2006), show that 1 to 3 grams of cinnamon powder daily can significantly improve blood-glucose control in adults with type 2 diabetes. The latest study, published in *Fertility & Sterility* (2007) examined oral cinnamon in adult women with polycystic ovary syndrome, a condition characterized by insulin resistance and a higher risk of acne. While they did not look at acne as an endpoint of the study, the researchers reported that 333 mg of cinnamon taken three times daily was effective in improving insulin resistance. Since cinnamon has recently been shown to be incredibly high in naturally occurring antioxidants, it certainly emerges as a candidate for inclusion in a clear skin diet. Scientists are hard at work trying to determine the specific components of cinnamon that make it so effective in stabilizing blood-glucose and insulin levels. PhytoMedical Technologies of Princeton, New Jersey, is a leader in this area and we hope they have a cinnamon-based product available in the not-too-distant future. Beyond the obvious application to diabetes, the cinnamon compounds should also be tried in acne research.

Excess Body Fat

There is now compelling evidence linking chronically elevated levels of insulin, insulin resistance, and elevated androgens with abdominal obesity. Such is certainly the case in polycystic ovary syndrome (PCO), which is associated with significant abdominal weight gain and, as mentioned, acne. The relationship between elevated androgens and abdominal obesity is not exclusive to PCO; a number of studies dating back to the early 80s have documented that even in healthy women, elevated androgens are associated with excess abdominal fat. A recent study from a group at Osijek University Hospital in Croatia showed that in healthy nondiabetic women, greater waist circumference (and not obesity per se) is associated with higher blood-insulin levels, insulin resistance, elevated testosterone, and less of those BPs that would otherwise decrease the biological activity of circulating testosterone. Abdominal weight gain is also associated with elevated C-reactive protein, the blood marker for inflammation. What is worse is that the fat cells (adipose tissue) are themselves generating androgens in women. Researchers from the University of Birmingham in the United Kingdom showed in 2004 that the androgen-converting enzyme 17β-HSD is alive and well in the fat cells of women, busy manufacturing testosterone. This, of course, helps explain why weight loss in women is associated with decreased testosterone levels.

Carrying excess body fat in the abdominal region is not associated with high levels of testosterone among males; here it is an elevation in the most potent "female" hormone, estradiol, which is associated with greater waist circumference. Given that 17β-HSD is involved in the manufacture of estradiol, and that 17β-HSD is active in fat cells, the elevated estradiol is not entirely surprising. In males, levels of the "female hormone" estradiol have been shown to be much higher in those with acne compared to those without. The reason is likely because of greater local conversion of testosterone to estradiol by an enzyme called aromatase. This enzyme is known to be very active in fat cells.

In both males and females, greater waist circumference is associated with increased markers of inflammation, increased generation of free radicals (oxidative stress), increased insulin and increased insulin resistance. It is also associated with elevated levels of the stress hormone cortisol, a finding we will discuss in more detail in chapter 6, "The Brain-Skin Connection." Research that did not evaluate body weight has shown that cortisol levels are elevated in both male and female acne patients.

Abdominal fat should be thought of as "active" tissue, a living organ with a busy work schedule. Far from lazy, these fat cells in the abdominal region should be considered workaholics. Not only does abdominal fat influence acne hormones, a recent study in the journal *Diabetes* (2005) showed that the abdominal fat cells also produce cortisol in significant quantities in humans. In addition, a research team from Osaka University in Japan found that increased oxidative stress within fat cells generates free radicals that have the potential to do damage throughout the body. Their important paper published in the *Journal of Clinical Investigation* (2004) suggests that carrying excess abdominal fat induces system-wide oxidative stress, and also that the oxidative stress inside fat cells causes abnormal secretion of chemical messengers from fat cells. Some of the chemical messengers released from fat cells include the immune chemicals called cytokines, which can promote inflammation.

It is certainly possible to be an extremely thin person and still have acne, and it is also evident that individuals who are overweight can have clear skin. Still, one might imagine that given the influences of fat cells on acne-promoting factors (e.g., hormones, oxidative stress, inflammation, cortisol), the chances of having acne as the waistline expands might be higher. It may once again come down to those genetic susceptibilities to acne and how environment can influence genetic expression. The first indication that this might be the case dates back to 1956 when researchers evaluated 2,730 military recruits and they found a significant relationship between acne and obesity in males twenty to forty years of age. This intriguing finding was never followed up until researchers from Taiwan published their findings in the *European Journal of Dermatology* (2006) after an investigation involving 3,274 schoolchildren evaluated for acne and body weight.

The researchers reported that the average body mass index (BMI) of students without acne was significantly lower than that of students with acne, and that those in the lowest BMI category had less overall acne and less inflammatory acne. For those in the upper BMI category, it was an opposite state of affairs.

The message seems pretty clear—maintaining a normal body weight and keeping abdominal fat off can decrease the risk of acne. Since the changes in hormones, oxidative stress, and inflammation reverse after improvement in body composition, a successful weight-loss endeavor may also diminish the severity of acne. The new Australian study published in the *Journal of the American Academy of Dermatology* (2007) did not note an association between weight loss and improvement of acne among young adults. Once again, it all comes down to genetic susceptibilities, so the clear skin diet high in whole grains, deeply colored fruits and vegetables, fish, and fiber, and low in processed foods, sugars, milk, animal-based saturated fats, and hydrogenated trans fats can influence genetics—and it also happens to be the diet most likely to keep your waistline from unwanted expansion.

No discussion of weight management can be complete without a mention of intentional physical activity—yes, exercise! The part of our bodies that burns the vast majority of calories is muscle. Ideal body composition means not only controlled body fat, it also means the maintenance of lean muscle mass. Most "weight-loss" diets result in a loss of both fat and its heavier counterpart—muscle. Retain and regain your muscle mass—combine a healthy diet with exercise and pay attention to waist size rather than weight per se. Remember that muscle weighs more than fat, so remind yourself that it is possible for your weight to remain unchanged to a great degree while your body composition improves.

Final Thoughts

Before moving on to the next chapter where we will explore the relationship between the gastrointestinal tract and acne, it's a good time to bring up a little historical commentary that was pretty much ignored in the dermatology community. It was April 1983, and dermatologist

Dr. William Kaufman of Sparks, Maryland, was calling for a proper investigation of dietary fiber as a means of influencing acne treatment outcome. He made note of the fact that proper gastrointestinal function was an important aspect of acne treatment in older dermatology textbooks. Writing in the *Archives of Dermatology*, he stated, "I believe correction of constipation is a favorable influence on acne . . . ," and went on to describe anecdotal reports of significant improvements after switching to an equivalent of ten additional grams of fiber at breakfast.

We now know that there are plausible biological mechanisms that would support Dr. Kaufman's anecdotal reports—the moderating influence of fiber on androgens, the prevention of insulin spikes in the blood, and the maintenance of healthy bacteria in the gastrointestinal tract, which can influence body-wide inflammation and oxidative stress (more on this in the next chapter). Refined grains, which, of course, are basically fiber-free, are stripped of important nutrients, the same nutrients that are deficient in those with acne. For example, compared to whole grain wheat flour, white flour contains 52 percent less selenium, and 75 percent less zinc. There is also no question that dietary fiber can aid in weight management. Higher fiber intake is associated with lower body weight and body fat, and fiber emerges as even more important than other nutrients with regard to BMI. Fiber allows us to eat more and weigh less because it displaces calorie-dense foods and makes you feel fuller. Simply put, fiber-rich foods are critical to the Clear Skin Diet.

Chapter Key Points

✔ Male hormones play a leading role in acne—they are made in the testes in males and the adrenal glands in both genders.

✔ Hormone and cancer risk may parallel hormone and acne risk.

✔ Dietary factors can influence testosterone.

✔ Testosterone decreases omega-3 DHA levels, and omega-3 fats can decrease testosterone levels. Saturated fats increase testosterone levels.

✔ Fiber raises sex-hormone-binding protein, and this in turn decreases free and active male hormones.

✔ Soy isoflavones and flavonoids from a long list of vegetables decrease oxidative stress and slow down the enzymes (5αR, 17β-HSD) that otherwise activate testosterone.

✔ Obesity is associated with acne risk, probably because it increases acne-related hormones, inflammation, and oxidative stress.

✔ Exercise is a critical component of a healthy lifestyle.

✔ Waist size is a better measure of ideal body composition, rather than simply total weight.

Acne—A Gut Reaction

W HY WOULD DERMATOLOGISTS WHO HAVE been trained that diet has no impact on acne concern themselves with intestinal function? How could this be of relevance to acne? After all, isn't intestinal function in the realm of the gastroenterologist anyway? Such has not always been the thinking, and if you do a little digging in the annals of acne treatment, you find that before the arrival of the wonder drugs, intestinal health was held in high regard when it came to acne patients. Dr. John H. Stokes et al.'s classic *Handbook of Fundamental Medical Dermatology* (1942) placed great emphasis on the management of a healthy GI tract and normal bowel movements.

Although we are born sterile, immediately after birth our gastrointestinal tract (GI) is colonized by a variety of bacteria. As life goes on, more and more bacteria will choose real estate in the intestines until as many as a trillion bacteria belonging to more than five hundred different species make up a crowded and vibrant environment. Most of the bacteria in a normal GI tract will reside in the colon (large intestine), with relatively few setting up camp in the small intestine. The collective intestinal bacteria are referred to as microflora, and healthy and normal microflora are now well known to play an important role in the promotion of human health. The bacteria that make up a healthy microflora have an enormous influence on the immune system, and they also secure the intestinal barrier, the "wall" that allows nutrients through and yet prevents toxins and unwanted materials from gaining access to the bloodstream.

Among the many bacterial genera that reside in the GI tract, there are two that are well recognized to be important in the promotion of health. *Lactobacilli* and *Bifidobacteria*, the so-called friendly bacteria that you might recognize from yogurt labels, are involved in vitamin synthesis, the detoxification and metabolism of toxic substances, stimulation of the immune response, protection from pathogenic (bad) bacteria, and the defense of the intestinal lining. In addition, *Lactobacilli* and *Bifidobacteria* can decrease oxidative stress and lower inflammation, locally in the gut as well as throughout the body. Recently, bacteria belonging to these genera have been shown to lower the levels of those inflammatory immune chemicals called cytokines, not only locally in the gut, but also body-wide when orally administered. This so-called "systemic" effect of the orally administered friendly bacteria is so pronounced that the oral administration of beneficial bacteria (aka probiotics) is capable of reducing *joint inflammation* in arthritic mammals!

The influence of the normal intestinal microflora has mostly been relegated to gut health, and it is only recently that researchers have been making some interesting connections with conditions that appear, at least on the surface, to have little to do with intestinal health. Some dermatologists were using tablets of probiotic *Lactobacillus* bacteria with reported success in the 1960s, yet in following with the same old theme in dermatology, this finding was never followed up, at least not in North America.

While Dr. John H. Stokes was advocating the use of *Lactobacillus* for general skin care in his 1942 textbook, Dr. Robert Siver, a dermatologist from Baltimore, was the first to formally report on the treatment of acne using probiotics (rather than antibiotics). He had originally been using *Lactobacillus* probiotics in cases with marked gastrointestinal disturbances and then he noticed a "side effect" of improved acne. This made him curious and he began to investigate the clinical value of *Lactobacillus* probiotics specifically for acne, regardless of gastrointestinal symptoms. Writing in *The Journal of the Medical Society of New Jersey* (1961), he reported significant value

of a *Lactobacillus* preparation called Lactinex. This preparation is still
on the market today and consists of two species of *Lactobacillus* bacteria—*Lactobacillus acidophilus* and *Lactobacillus bulgaricus*—with a total
of one million bacteria (referred to as colony-forming units or cfu)
per tablet. Dr. Siver reported on three hundred patients with acne
who were administered two or three tablets three times daily for eight
days. This was followed by two weeks without the probiotics, and
then readministration of the probiotics for another eight days. The
protocol was reported to be very effective, with only 20 percent of the
patients showing no response. Of the 80 percent who did respond, the
majority showed benefit during the first course, although for some,
positive results were noted after three months. The Lactinex was most
effective in treating inflammatory acne and appeared to be most valuable to younger patients who had not been the subject of prolonged
conventional therapies. Dr. Siver states in the journal: "*Lactobacillus* is
not a universal cure for acne. . . . However, clinical experience suggests
involvement of the metabolic products present in the preparation
[Lactinex] and associated with the gastrointestinal tract. Interactions
of skin manifestations of acne vulgaris and of metabolic processes of
the intestinal tract are suggestive."

Dr. Siver was onto something; he had no idea that sophisticated
research in the late 1990s and in the first years of the new millennium
would indeed show that the metabolic processes of the intestinal tract
and its resident bacteria have untold influences on areas far removed
from the colon. His preliminary investigations with probiotics sat
dormant until Italian researchers stepped up twenty-six years later
with a two-month study involving probiotics added to standard acne
therapy. The research, published in *La Clinica Terapeutica* (1987),
examined forty patients ages fourteen to thirty-three, all of whom
were given the standard acne therapy of the day—antibiotics, benzoyl peroxide, retinol, and anti-androgen medications. The only difference was that one group also received an encapsulated probiotic
preparation containing 250 mg of freeze-dried *Lactobacillus acidophilus*
and *Bifidobacteria bifidum*. The probiotic capsules were taken three
times per day on an empty stomach for the course of the two-month
study. In the end, those who were in the probiotic group had marked
improvements in acne relative to those without the probiotics, par-

ticularly in the area of comedo formation and inflammatory, cystic lesions. None of the patients in the probiotic group experienced side effects from probiotic preparation; in fact, they tolerated the prescribed antibiotics quite well—such was not the case in the group without the probiotic, where intolerance to the antibiotics was reported by a number of patients.

Once again, things were quiet until Russian researcher Dr. L. A. Volkova and colleagues from the Center for Medical Cosmetology in Moscow reported on the intestinal microflora of acne patients and the benefit of probiotics. They found that the majority of patients with acne (54 percent) had marked alterations in the bacteria that make up the intestinal microflora. It really didn't matter if the acne was more cystic or more pustular; inflammatory acne was associated with an altered microflora in most patients. Just as Dr. Francesco Marchetti and colleagues from Italy had done in 1987, the Russian doctors added a mixture of probiotics to the standard care of acne. Writing in the Russian journal *Klinicheskaia Meditsina* (2001), the researchers reported that when they added probiotics to the regimen of standard care among those with alterations of the intestinal microflora, there were significant improvements and a more rapid resolution of acne lesions compared to standard care alone.

Microbes populate the skin as well as the gut, albeit in much smaller numbers and in an environment that is drier and well oxygenated. The inhabitants, as you might imagine, are therefore somewhat different from those on the inside. Topical application of probiotics might have some potential, although to date there has been little research. In one recent study, researchers from the Division of Food Science, Korea University, reported that a natural chemical produced by *Lactococcus* HY449 may be beneficial as a topical treatment for acne. An antimicrobial chemical secreted by this probiotic called bacteriocin proved to be toxic to the bacteria involved in acne— *Propionibacterium acnes*. A second study showed that five dairy-derived variants of *Propionibacteria* can suppress the growth of bacteria that cause skin infections. It appeared that the organic acids they manufacture are responsible for this antimicrobial influence against less desirable bacteria. The point is that we can use bacteria to fight bacteria. We hope probiotics and/or probiotic components will prove to be useful and will be available for topical use in the not-too-distant future. In the meantime, orally administered probiotic strains may be important, have an excellent safety profile, and should not be over-looked. Antibiotics wreak havoc on the GI tract by clear-cutting the resident beneficial bacteria, and eventually the overuse of antibiotics leads to microbial resistance—this means that when we really need antibiotics to work for lifesaving situations, they may be ineffective against pathogenic (bad) bacteria.

Why shouldn't we treat acne with antibiotics? There are three good reasons. First, acne is not primarily a condition defined by infec-tion. In early treatment, before colonization with *P. acnes*, antibiotic therapy is not warranted. The second reason is that they tend to stop working after a few to several months. This happens because the *P. acnes* become resistant to the antimicrobial effects. Of course, we can just switch to a different antibiotic, and many dermatologists find themselves and their patients on this merry-go-round, getting off one and jumping on another. Sadly, *P. acnes* is not the only microbe that is flexing its muscles and developing resistance. Our normal bacte-rial residents tend to become resistant, and they, in turn, can pass on the resistance factor to disease-causing bacteria. The practice of overusing antibiotics has resulted in so-called "superbugs" which are multi-resistant. We need to remain cognizant of the fact that it is not just the acne patient (or the recipient of the antibiotic) who has the potential to develop this resistance problem—for reasons that are not entirely clear, the members of the patient's household also show the same resistance patterns without actually taking antibiotics!

A third problem with long-term antibiotic treatment, as mentioned above, is the consequence of "clear-cutting" the normal bacterial resi-dents of the gut, vagina, and skin itself. These more-friendly bacteria are also killed off in the process of attacking the "bad" bacteria. Yeast overgrowth, particularly yeast vaginitis, is a universally recognized side effect of oral antibiotics. Overgrowth of *Malassezia* yeast in acne patients is much more common than usually recognized. Antibiotic-associated diarrhea is not rare; it can occur in up to 25 percent of patients, depending on the medication. Two recent reports should give frequent antibiotic prescribers cause for serious concern. A study published in the *Journal of the American Medical Association* (2004) showed a link between antibiotic use and breast cancer. Following this, researchers from the University of Pennsylvania reported in the *Archives of Dermatology* (2005) that acne patients taking oral antibiotics were more likely to experience upper respiratory infections than those who did not take antibiotics.

A final area of concern with the use of antibiotic medications is the environmental impact. Dr. Ettore Zuccato and colleagues reported in *Lancet* (2000) that thousands of tons of pharmaceutical drugs are excreted by humans and animals that consume them, some as active components that escape degradation in waste management. Erythromycin, an antibiotic used in acne treatment, can persist in the environment for more than a year. Researchers attempted to detect sixteen commonly prescribed drugs in Italian river water samples and were able to find measurable amounts of fourteen! The concentrations may have been too low to have medicinal effects; however, what about the unknown of lifetime exposure in the entire food chain, including aquatic organisms? Similar findings have been reported in North America. As stated by U.S. Environmental Protection Agency scientist Dr. Christian G. Daughton in *Lancet* (2002), there is a "critical need for collaboration between the traditionally separated environmental and medical sciences."

The overprescribing of antibiotics is appalling. At one time antibiotics were prescribed like candies, and although things have improved, they are still grossly overused. As we discussed in chapter 1, antibiotics are now being associated with the onset of a number of human conditions, including irritable bowel syndrome, Crohn's disease, breast cancer, allergies, upper respiratory tract infections, and asthma. The common thread among all of these conditions is documented alterations in intestinal and nasal microflora. Up to 85 percent of antibiotic prescriptions for sore throats, coughs, and colds are unwarranted. The long-term disruption of normal intestinal microflora by antibiotics is well known, but only recently has the importance of maintaining a healthy gut microflora been given scientific support. Antibiotics should be reserved for the times when they are really needed, and if the overprescribing is not curtailed, they will be much less likely to work when we need them. The issue of antibiotic resistance by smart bacteria is becoming a global concern.

Probiotic Mechanisms in Acne

The exact mechanisms behind the benefits of friendly gut bacteria such as *Lactobacillus* and *Bifidobacteria* are unknown; however, we can speculate on some potential pathways related to acne. The body-wide anti-inflammatory and antioxidant effects of oral probiotics have now been demonstrated in a number of studies. Since inflammation and oxidative stress are two consistent features of acne, it is not entirely surprising that various international investigators have reported successful outcomes with probiotics.

A remarkable study in the *Journal of Nutrition* (2004) showed that the effect of administering commercially available *Lactobacillus GG* was so significant that it reduced redness and swelling in the joints of arthritic animals. Interestingly, plain yogurt fermented with typical *Lactobacillus*-based starter culture did have a mild to moderate anti-inflammatory effect, while regular milk had no benefit at all. Probiotics are capable of influencing the inflammatory-immune chemicals to an impressive degree, and this is the likely mechanism behind the anti-inflammatory activities.

Recent studies also show that species of the *Lactobacillus* and *Bifidobacteria* genera act as major antioxidants. At least four studies have shown that probiotics are protective against free-radical damage, particularly against damage to the lipid (fat) component of cells. In one eye-opening study by Dr. Tatyana Oxman and colleagues from Israel, *orally* administered *Lactobacillus bulgaricus* was shown to protect heart cells against the effects of ischemia (lack of oxygenated blood supply). The protective effects were most likely related to an antioxidant effect. The studies are not limited only to test tubes and animals, a few have looked at the broad antioxidant activity of probiotics in humans as well; in one study, published in the *American Journal of Clinical Nutrition* (2003), Swedish researchers showed that a strain of *Lactobacillus plantarum*, identified as 299V, could improve cardiovascular risk factors in adult smokers. Specifically, they showed that oral administration of the bacteria lowered blood pressure, inflammatory cytokines, and free radical blood markers associated with cardiovascular disease. There was also a 37 percent reduction in reliable blood markers of oxidative stress, markers that are typically elevated in a variety of chronic diseases. In addition, the *Lactobacillus plantarum* 299V group had a 42 percent reduction in blood levels of the inflammatory cytokine IL-6, which may play an important role in acne. This excellent strain of bacteria is well suited for acne patients and is now commercially available as LactoFlamX from Metagenics Inc. (see the appendix).

Following this, a study in *Nutrition Journal* (2005) showed that oral administration of *Lactobacillus fermentum* ME-3 capsules (versus a placebo) boosted blood antioxidant strength and improved overall antioxidant status in a group of healthy adults forty to sixty years of age. This type of evidence makes it very clear that the bacteria residing in the intestinal tract can have far-reaching effects, way beyond the gut. It truly is amazing that collectively these tiny microbes are capable of lowering oxidative stress and inflammatory chemicals outside the gut.

Consider also a study in the *American Journal of Clinical Nutrition* (2003), where it was demonstrated that consumption of commercially available *Lactobacillus GG* capsules was capable of lowering the levels of undesirable, infection-causing bacteria in the nasal cavity. Separate studies have indicated that taking probiotics and yogurts with live active bacterial cultures (including *Lactobacillus*) by mouth can positively influence vaginal microflora, cutting the risk of infection in women. It is therefore entirely possible that orally administered probiotics may influence the resident skin bacteria. The more we learn about these tiny microbes that we have been systematically wiping out with acne antibiotics, the more we realize that we still haven't scratched the surface of how they help us. Long-term treatment of acne patients with antibiotics such as tetracyclines has been shown to influence the microflora of household relatives as well. Family members of similar age who live together (e.g., spouses) quite often have a near identical makeup of intestinal microflora. The reasons for this are not well understood; however, diet and environment are probably big players. Research from more than two decades ago, published in the *Journal of Investigative Dermatology* (1985), shows that antibiotic administration to acne patients for a little over one year caused an expected increase in antibiotic-resistant organisms among the acne patients. This is bad enough; however, what was really alarming was that the nontreated household relatives—those who never even touched an antibiotic for the course of the fourteen months—also developed antibiotic-resistant strains in a similar pattern to the antibiotic-treated patients. So taking long-term oral antibiotics can influence the microflora of family members as well, and how it happens remains a mystery. As mentioned, the more we learn about the microbes that have peacefully coexisted in and on us for centuries, the more we realize that we don't know much at all.

Dietary Influences on Microflora

We are beginning to get a handle on how diet can influence the levels of the friendly bacteria that reside in the GI tract. Consider Japan, a place where rates of acne were half those of North America just a few decades ago, before the rapid Westernization of the Japanese diet took place in the 1980s and 1990s. If diet does indeed influence microflora, then one might imagine differences between Japanese adults and North American adults consuming radically different diets might be evident upon testing. In 1986, researchers from the University of Tokyo and the Ludwig Institute of Cancer in Toronto compared the fecal microflora of Japanese residents consuming a typical Japanese diet to that of healthy Torontonians consuming a typical Western diet. As you may have guessed, the levels of *Lactobacillus* and *Bifidobacteria* were significantly higher among the Japanese. In contrast, the Canadians had much higher levels of the *Bacteroides* (suspected in cancer) and various *Clostridium* species (bacteria suspected in autism).

The Japanese diet contains elements known to promote the growth of friendly intestinal microflora. Take, for example, green tea, which we discussed as having great potential in the treatment of acne. Research shows that green tea promotes the growth of *Bifidobacteria*, and, surprisingly, the most likely antiacne component within green tea, EGCG, has been shown to enhance the effectiveness of antifungal medications against yeasts in the gut. In fact, the most pronounced effect of EGCG from green tea was against undesirable microbes, including the drug-resistant *Candida* strains. In addition to its antioxidant and anti-inflammatory activities, ginger has also been reported to have strong antimicrobial properties, yet it appears to stimulate the growth of *Lactobacillus*. Honey in moderation is a great way to naturally sweeten foods because it contains antioxidant polyphenols, and at least two studies have shown that it can selectively promote the growth of *Bifidobacteria* and *Lactobacillus*. The dietary fiber we discussed, the omega-3 fatty acids from fish, the green tea, and a host of other colorful phytonutrients within the Japanese diet may influence intestinal microflora in a beneficial way.

Even within Japan, adherence to a higher-fiber traditional diet can influence the intestinal bacteria. In an eye-opening study published in *Applied and Environmental Microbiology* (1989), researchers from the University of Tokyo showed that those living in the rural Yuzurihara/Yamanashi regions had a different intestinal microflora profile from those living in urban Tokyo. What was so special about this was that the Yuzurihara/Yamanashi regions include the residences of some of the longest-lived individuals in Japan, and they adhere more closely to the traditional Japanese diet compared to their cosmopolitan counterparts in Tokyo. The overall levels of *Bifidobacteria* were much higher in the rural, long-lived regions than in Tokyo. In addition, there were much lower levels of the problematic *Clostridium* and *Bacteroides* groups. The loss of *Bifidobacteria* and a gain in the *Clostridium* and *Bacteroides* groups can increase fermentation and formation of less desirable, even toxic, protein breakdown products.

The traditional Japanese diet is of course rich in omega-3 fatty acids derived from fish and seafood. In addition to their anti-inflammatory role, omega-3 fatty acids may also be promoting a healthy gut microflora. Research shows that all types of dietary fats do not have the same effect when it comes to influencing the growth of intestinal bacteria. Japanese researchers showed that among three different diets (one high in omega-6 corn oil, another high in beef fat, and a third high in fish oil), it was the group supplemented with fish oil that showed a beneficial effect on intestinal flora. In fact, the fish-oil diet led to a threefold increase in *Bifidobacteria* and the lowest levels of the *Bacteroides* group of bacteria. This is significant because *Bacteroides* are implicated in cancer. In a separate study, it was shown that a diet high in fish oil or flaxseed oil, both rich in omega-3, can increase *Lactobacillus* growth. In contrast, coconut oil, high in saturated fats, did not increase beneficial bacteria. In addition, experimental studies have shown that omega-6–rich corn oil and pure linoleic acid itself (parent omega-6 oil) are both *inhibitory* to the growth of *Bifidobacteria*. Pure EPA from fish oil, on the other hand, is inhibitory to human *Bacteroides.*

Beyond the increase in the growth of beneficial bacteria, the polyunsaturated fats appear to influence the adhesion of good bacteria to the intestinal wall. Arachidonic acid is found in beef fat, and it is also produced from those omega-6 vegetable oils (corn, soybean, safflower, sunflower) we are overconsuming. Arachidonic acid, the main promoter of the inflammatory acne chemicals PGE2 and LTB4, also causes less adhesion of good bacteria to intestinal cells. In contrast, flaxseed oil, rich in omega-3, increases the adhesion of friendly bacteria to the cells that make up the intestinal wall. Marine oils, high in EPA, have been shown to markedly increase the adhesion of *Lactobacillus* to the intestines.

Published reports from as far back as 1964 have shown that olive oil can increase numbers of *Lactobacillus*. Researchers are just now beginning to understand how different lipids might influence the adhesion of bacteria. Astonishingly, these fatty acids are actually taken up inside the bacteria, and this, in turn, can change the shape of the "body" or structure of the bacteria—this change in bacterial shape is then responsible for alterations in the adhesion (or stickiness) to the cells of the intestinal wall. So far, the preponderance of evidence suggests that our overconsumption of omega-6 fatty acids (and underconsumption of omega-3) might be having a negative impact on our gut microflora.

The relationship between omega-3 fatty acids and friendly bacteria is a symbiotic one that appears to also run in the opposite direction—probiotics might also influence omega-3 status. When researchers from Finland investigated the administration of oral *Bifidobacteria* to allergic children, not only did they find benefit, they also noted an increase in the parent omega-3 fatty acid, alpha-linolenic acid. Further hints come from a McGill University study where hens fed a *Lactobacillus* probiotic blend mixed into flaxseed had higher levels of EPA in eggs than hens fed flax-based food alone. So that old saying "You are what you eat" should really be updated to "You are what what you *eat*, eats"!

The Brassica Family of Vegetables		
arugula	cauliflower	purple cauliflower
bok choy	Chinese broccoli	radish
broccoli	daikon	rutabaga
broccoli sprouts	horseradish	wasabi
broccolini	kale	watercress
Brussels sprouts	kohlrabi	
cabbage	mustard greens	

Another group of foods that can positively influence intestinal microflora is the vegetable family known as "the great cleansers"—the *Brassica* family of vegetables. *Brassica* foods appear to have selective effects on intestinal microbial inhabitants. Broccoli sprouts and wasabi, in particular, are known inhibitors of the nasty stomach bacteria *Helicobacter pylori*, the one involved in the formation of ulcers. Yet, wasabi and broccoli sprouts appear to leave *Lactobacillus* and *Bifidobacteria* alone.

As mentioned in the last chapter, chronic constipation has been associated, at least anecdotally, with acne for many decades. The relationship between a sluggish bowel and skin conditions including acne has been hanging around for a long time; even the ancient Egyptians suggested that a toxic agent associated with the feces was related to disease. Improper elimination of the bowels was thought to lead to something called intestinal "autointoxication." The term autointoxication, coined more than one hundred years ago, refers to the notion that a variety of diseases can arise from toxins produced within the gastrointestinal tract. In the 1800s, with the advancement of science, some theorized that the decomposition of proteins in the intestines (termed "putrefaction") could cause illness and disease. The staunch proponents of autointoxication did go a little overboard in the early part of the twentieth century, when it was proposed that constipation was the root of almost all illness, and some surgeons even suggested just cutting out the colon to prevent everything from skin wrinkling to dementia.

Elie Metchnikoff, winner of the 1908 Nobel Prize of Medicine, also suggested that health was compromised due to toxins from the gut, and his solution was to alter the intestinal microflora by introducing more friendly bacteria. He came to this conclusion after examining the diets of the Bulgarians, the Turks, and the Armenians, who had notable health and longevity. Among the three diets, the frequent consumption of fermented milk was the common thread. He identified two bacteria in fermented milk, *Lactobacillus bulgaricus* and *Streptococcus thermophilus*. These were held to improve bowel function, prevent the accumulation of toxins, and improve overall health. A clear complexion was one aspect of health that became closely tied to gastrointestinal health, and the subsequent inclusion of proper bowel functioning as a means to address acne in dermatology textbooks was based more on the clinical experience and anecdotes of the time.

Constipation and acne have never been scientifically evaluated; however, based on new research published in the journal *Digestive and Liver Disease* (2005), we now know that chronic constipation is indeed associated with significant changes in the intestinal microflora. As you probably guessed, there are lower beneficial *Lactobacillus* and *Bifidobacteria* levels and a disturbing increase in intestinal permeability (inappropriately porous gastrointestinal barrier). Chronic constipation is also associated with an elevation in body-wide immune system activity (i.e., chronic constipation is provoking an unnecessary, inflammatory immune response beyond the reaches of the local GI tract). The low-grade inflammatory response could be due in part to unwanted materials' gaining body-wide access through a more permeable intestinal tract. Given that chronic low-grade inflammation is a major player in many chronic medical conditions including acne, the importance of this new research cannot be overstated. This may also explain why the older dermatology texts were so keen on ensuring normal bowel functioning in acne patients.

New research has also allowed us to see that specific bacteria within the intestinal tract can influence the motility (or propulsion) of food and waste matter through the GI tract. Researchers have shown that *Lactobacillus* and *Bifidobacteria* actually speed things up and promote the transit of material through the intestines. *E. coli*, on the other hand, bacteria that can ferment proteins and produce toxic chemicals, actually slows down movement. With this background, it would seem plausible that the oral delivery of probiotic strains might improve constipation. In a landmark study in the *Canadian Journal of Gastroenterology* (2003), researchers showed that *Lactobacillus casei* strain Shirota has a highly significant effect toward improving chronic constipation. Compared to a placebo, the *Lactobacillus casei* Shirota (consumed as a beverage called Yakult) group showed significant improvement in both stool consistency and bowel movements. Positive effects were noted about two weeks into the one-month study. It was reported that 89 percent of those in the Yakult group experienced improvement in constipation, which was almost double that of the placebo group.

Stress and Intestinal Bacteria

Most patients with acne consider stress to be a strong provocateur of the illness, and modern research has backed up this assumption. A large body of research has also shown that psychological and physical stressors have a considerable negative impact on the beneficial intestinal bacteria. Actually, stress might be considered a potent antibiotic against the good *Lactobacillus* and *Bifidobacteria*. The first reports that stress could impact the intestinal flora came in the late 1970s when researchers showed states of anger and fear can increase potentially negative *Bacteroides theta* by almost tenfold. Interestingly, they found that this type of emotional response increased the specific strain of *Bacteroides* that has been linked with obesity. As reported recently in *Discover* (2005), researchers from the Karolinska Institute have found that *Bacteroides theta* promotes abdominal fat storage. This research suggests that weight gain associated with stress may be, at least in part, directed by alterations in our intestinal microflora.

Following this, Russian investigators reported on studies they had been conducting with a group of cosmonauts who were preparing for flight. In the days leading up to the launch, as nervous emotional stressors became higher, there were marked decreases in *Lactobacillus* and *Bifidobacteria*. It was the *Bifidobacteria* that appeared to be extremely vulnerable to preflight emotional stress. Even after the flight, however, the microflora remained altered, with increases in less-desirable *Clostridia* species and significant decreases in *Lactobacillus* and *Bifidobacteria*.

Endurance athletes are well known to have gastrointestinal complaints. One study showed that endurance athletes who train intensively for about two hours every day have lower levels of *Bifidobacteria*. The athletes who work to near exhaustion may have gastrointestinal complaints due to stress-induced alterations in the intestinal microflora. There are numerous reports from animal studies that indicate stress can alter the intestinal microflora. Overcrowding and excessive heat can increase less-desirable bacteria and decrease *Lactobacillus*. Noise stress and a feeling of being trapped will lower *Lactobacillus* in laboratory animals. Psychological stress encourages the growth of yeasts in animals—an overgrowth that can be inhibited with the anti-anxiety medication Xanax. In other words, taking a drug that helps curb the stress reaction can limit changes in the intestinal microflora. Researchers showed that there were marked increases in *Candida* species within the intestines among those who survived the devastating 1995 Hanshin-Awaji earthquake in Japan. Higher *Candida* levels were noted in subjects who lived closer to severely earthquake-damaged areas, indicating a connection to higher stress levels.

The effects of intestinal bacteria may even extend to human behavior itself. Among primates, maternal stress during pregnancy can result in a reduction of both *Lactobacillus* and *Bifidobactera* concentrations. In the offspring, measures of infant independence are correlated with infant *Lactobacillus* and *Bifidobacteria*. In other words, the infant primates with higher *Lactobacillus* and *Bifidobacteria* species were more independent and exploratory than those with low levels of friendly bacteria. Lower *Lactobacillus* levels have been specifically correlated with the display of stress-indicative behaviors in animals. Interestingly, maternal anxiety and depression have been tied to a higher risk of infantile colic in the offspring. Infants who experience colic have been documented to have lower levels of intestinal *Lactobacillus*, and a recent study in the journal *Pediatrics* (2007) shows that oral administration of a commercially available probiotic strain (*Lactobacillus reuteri*) improves infantile colic.

The reason for the stress and good-bacteria connection is not known for sure, but it may have do with changes in intestinal motility, or the direct effects of stress chemicals. Research published in the *World Journal of Gastroenterology* (2005) showed that psychological stress interferes with the movement of food through the GI tract and causes overgrowth of unwanted bacteria in the small intestine that block the absorption of nutrients. In addition to the stress-related reductions in *Lactobacillus*, psychological stress also makes the intestine more permeable to undesirable material. Whatever the cause of stress-induced alterations to the intestinal microflora, it is clear that the consumption of probiotic bacteria may be advisable during times of stress. We will explore the stress-acne connection in more detail in the next chapter.

Probiotics

A joint team from the United Nations Food and Agriculture Organization and the World Health Organization defined probiotics in 2002 as live microorganisms (bacteria, yeast, etc.) which, when administered in adequate amounts, confer a beneficial effect on the host. The route of administration was not specified, although most often they are taken by mouth. The benefit is not limited to the GI tract, something we have been emphasizing in this chapter—the potential value can be observed well beyond the confines of gastroenterology.

A recent review in the *Journal of Clinical Gastroenterology* (2005) highlighted the evidence for probiotics in human health. Researchers from Yale University and the University of Connecticut identified 288 health-related outcomes in human clinical trials published from 1980 through August 2004. Remarkably, they found that there were 239 positive outcomes noted, and only 49 negative or no-effect results. The vast majority of the studies used just a single strain of bacteria, while only sixty used multiple bacterial strains. Among the results, ten outcome measurements examined certain strains of bacteria on lactose intolerance—in eight of these ten outcome measurements, probiotics positively influenced lactose intolerance. The bottom line is that there is research supporting probiotics, but probiotics are certainly not all alike, and the specific strain of the bacteria may be important.

Dr. Martin Katzman is a psychiatrist at the University of Toronto who, along with Dr. Logan, has generated a hypothesis that probiotics might influence brain/behavior, even depressive symptoms. Their findings were formally published in the journal *Medical Hypotheses* (2005), where they speculated that the ability of probiotics to communicate with the nervous system, influence oxidative stress, inflammation, gut function, and overall nutritional status might make these friendly bacteria of interest in mood regulation. In other words, because probiotics confer so many health benefits to the host (humans), some of which influence the nervous system, the result of consumption might influence daily mood. In a placebo-controlled study published in the *European Journal of Clinical Nutrition* (2006), Dr. David Benton and colleagues confirmed that probiotics can influence mood, at least in some individuals. They found that Yakult, the same fermented dairy beverage shown to improve constipation, consumed daily led to significant improvements in mood states among healthy adults who had poor baseline self-reported mood. The fermented beverage did little if the mood was already in the higher range at baseline; however, it made a big difference in those who had initially scored low on the Profile of Mood States scale. Hopefully, further research will determine if Yakult (*Lactobacillus casei* strain Shirota) or other quality probiotics can influence the psychological fallout and the direct causes of acne.

Despite the potential benefits, one of the most significant problems with probiotics is finding a brand that has therapeutic levels of viable bacteria within the capsule, powder, food, or beverage. There have been a number of reports in the United States, Canada, and Europe where independent testing has revealed that there are few, if any, live bacteria in commercial pills, powders, and yogurts. In addition, the beneficial effects of probiotics appear to be specific to the strain of bacteria involved. It is disturbing that probiotics are still marketed under the umbrella term "acidophilus," and consumers are led to believe that any old probiotic (or acidophilus!) will do. The research shows otherwise, and consumers should know that there are three important parts to a probiotic name—genus, species, and strain. For example, two of the more researched strains in the world are *Lactobacillus* (genus) *casei* (species) Shirota (strain) and *Lactobacillus* (genus) *plantarum* (species) 299V (strain). These are well-documented bacterial strains that have been the subject of scientific and medical research.

We think it is important to point out that there are also so-called "prebiotics" that are commercially available. These are nondigestible food ingredients such as fructo-oligosaccharides (FOS) that are basically food for intestinal bacteria. In several well-controlled animal studies, researchers have shown that prebiotics, and FOS in particular, can lead to a more porous intestinal wall, resulting in bad bacteria such as Salmonella getting through the intestinal wall and causing some major problems. FOS can cause significant gut-wall inflammation, and in the latest study in the *Journal of Nutrition* (2006), researchers confirmed that indeed FOS causes flatulence, intestinal bloating, and appears to irritate the gut lining, potentially influencing intestinal barrier-wall function in adults. Based on this emerging research, it is difficult to support the use of stand-alone prebiotic products or yogurts that are using significant quantities of prebiotic.

See the appendix for recommended probiotics.

Chapter Key Points

✔ We have more than a trillion microbes living in our intestines.

✔ "Good" microbes synthesize vitamins, break down toxins, support immune function, protect against "bad"/infectious microbes, and defend the lining of the intestine.

✔ Probiotics in foods or supplements are live "good" bacteria or yeasts that have a beneficial effect for us.

✔ There may be an altered profile of the resident "good" bacteria in the intestines of acne patients.

✔ Preliminary studies from the United States, Italy, and Russia have shown value in acne treatment when oral probiotic bacteria are added to conventional care.

✔ While the microenvironment of the skin differs from that of the gut, "good" bacteria also inhabit the skin.

✔ Preliminary research suggests potential in acne for the topical application of probiotics and/or the natural chemicals they secrete.

✔ There are compelling reasons to curb antibiotic prescriptions for acne—lack of long-term efficacy, development of resistance against antibiotics, increasing the population of unwanted yeasts, elimination of "good" bacteria, and environmental pollution.

6

The Brain-Skin Connection

THE SKIN AND THE BRAIN seem so far removed from each other that it is difficult to imagine there would be major physiological links between the two. Yet, scientists are just now uncovering the true depth of the relationship between the brain and our skin. Right from the start of our existence, they both grow up together because the nervous system and skin share the same embryological origin, a collection of cells called the embryonic ectoderm. The skin and central nervous system share similar hormones and neurotransmitters (chemical messengers) that work like a key opening up a high security lock to bring about physiological changes.

Recently, scientists have discovered that the skin itself is capable of manufacturing many chemicals once thought to be exclusive to the brain and nervous system. Researchers from Toyama Medical University in Japan have shown that nerves once thought to regulate only bodily pain are indeed innervating the sebaceous glands! These nerves release a chemical called substance P, which in turn stimulates sebum production. Psychological stress and anxiety are associated with enhanced substance P release; on the other hand, relaxation therapies including massage therapy have been associated with a reduction of substance P levels. These exciting new findings on the relationship between the nervous system and the pilosebaceous unit might at least partially explain the long-held notion of a stress-acne connection. It may also shed light on other stress-related skin conditions including seborrheic dermatitis and acne rosacea.

The emotional impact of acne on the individual can be profound. Acne can lead to major problems with self-esteem, social functioning, and self-confidence. Since the face is most often the site of acne presentation, and facial appearance is highly linked to body image, it is not difficult to imagine that the experience of acne is extremely stressful. The psychological fallout manifests as embarrassment, social withdrawal, depression, anxiety, anger, and, ultimately, impaired social functioning. This, in turn, translates into poorer academic achievement, less interaction with members of the opposite sex, decreased participation in sports, and, according to one study in the United Kingdom, a 70 percent higher unemployment rate among those with acne.

Experienced dermatologists are well aware that acne is not a trivial teen disease that simply passes in time with little consequence. As stated a half century ago in the *Medical Clinics of North America* (1948), "There is no single disease that causes more psychic trauma, more maladjustment between parents and children, and more general insecurity and feelings of inferiority, and greater sums of psychic suffering than does acne vulgaris." The depth of acne suffering was made a little clearer in 1999, when researchers from Oxford University in the United Kingdom discovered that the social, psychological, and emotional problems of acne patients are even worse than many prevalent and disabling chronic diseases. The mental health scores for acne patients ages sixteen to thirty-nine were worse than those with asthma, epilepsy, diabetes, back pain, coronary artery disease, or arthritis.

More recently, a team from New Zealand reported in the *Journal of Paediatrics and Child Health* (2006) that there is an urgent need to attend to the mental health of teens with acne. These investigators worked with almost ten thousand students ages twelve to eighteen and determined that "problem acne" was associated with a more than twofold risk of depression and anxiety. They also found that the teens with so-called problem acne were almost twice as likely to have made a suicide attempt.

Despite this well-documented relationship between acne and

psychological impairment, the experience of acne is still trivialized outside the dermatology community. Medical conditions perceived as trivial or unimportant become marginalized when it comes to scientific research. Sadly, even though acne patients may be worse off psychologically than those with many other chronic diseases, the acne-stress research is like a tiny minnow compared to other conditions.

While acne causes psychological discomfort in most patients to some degree or another, in many cases it can be associated with clinically significant, diagnosable anxiety and depression. Various studies show that about 30 percent of patients with acne are clinically depressed, and a further 44 percent have clinically significant anxiety. Patients with acne are up to two times more likely to have body dysmorphic disorder, a condition characterized by a disturbed body image. As mentioned, thoughts of and attempts at suicide are also much higher among acne patients. Anger is closely linked with acne, and indeed even with the severity of acne lesions. Research indicates that the psychological impact on adult acne patients may be even more severe, probably because society tells us that acne should be gone before the twentieth birthday. Overall, the incidence of emotional disorders in acne patients is twice that of the general population.

By and large, there has been an assumption that the psychological fallout, the depression, the anxiety and anger, all are a result of actually experiencing acne itself. It is certainly a reasonable assumption, and most acne patients would also agree that acne takes a significant emotional toll. However, as nutritional doctors, we also wonder about the contrary perspective, that individuals who experience acne suffer higher risk for depression, anxiety, and anger due to overlapping nutritional inadequacies. In other words, what if the same nutritional influences on depression, anger, and other mood alterations are also at work in acne? Maybe the higher rates of depression, anxiety, and anger should be expected to emerge among acne patients because deficiencies of omega-3 fatty acids, zinc, selenium, magnesium, dietary fiber, vitamin A, and other antioxidants have all been linked to depressed mood and even suicide. We now know that the same inadequate omega-3 fatty acid intake and lack of fiber and dietary antioxidants that combine to promote cardiovascular disease are also playing a role in depressive and behavioral disorders. We know that serious cardiovascular disease is life-altering and can limit an individual's life—yet it is those who experience deep depression as a result of cardiovascular disease who are at most risk of dying. It is also true that those with both cardiovascular disease and depression have the lowest levels of omega-3 fatty acids. Those same nutritional voids and reliance upon processed, calorie-dense, nutritionally poor foods are likely to account for the higher risk of cardiovascular disease in those who have experienced depression in early life. Our theory is that those who experience depression and anxiety in early life will be at greater risk of acne over the course of a lifetime, and that the nutritional factors that overlap between mental health and acne are the common thread between the two.

Emerging research reveals that the relationship between nutrition and mental health has been grossly underappreciated. A host of laboratory, experimental, and large-population studies have shown that low omega-3 levels are associated with altered mood states, anger, and depression. Since the brain itself is 60 percent fat, it should not be shocking that omega-3 fatty acids have emerged as being important for both brain-cell structure and function. The omega-3 fatty acid docosahexaenoic acid (DHA) makes up a significant portion of the nerve cell wall, while the anti-inflammatory omega-3 eicosapentaenoic acid (EPA), which holds great promise in treating acne, is responsible for communication within and among nerve cells.

There are several lines of scientific evidence that connect omega-3 fatty acid intake and various forms of depression. More than a few studies have shown that fish and seafood consumption appears to be protective against depression, seasonal affective disorder (so-called winter blues), bipolar (manic) depression, and postpartum depression. Dr. Joseph Hibbeln and colleagues from the National Institutes of Health have been looking into this area of research for well over a decade. His team has consistently shown that higher fish and seafood consumption is associated with lower rates of depressive conditions. Australian and European researchers have also shown that even within a country, greater intake of fish is associated with a lower risk of depression and higher overall mental health status.

More than a half dozen intervention studies using fish oil, and

EPA in particular, have shown that marine-derived omega-3 fatty acids can improve depressive symptoms in adults with depressive disorders. However, the benefits of taking fish oil may also be apparent in healthy adults, as research in the *European Journal of Clinical Investigation* (2005) showed that one month of fish oil (versus olive oil) supplementation improved both mood and mental functioning in otherwise healthy adults. Then in December 2005, Dr. Laure Buydens and colleagues reported that EPA-rich fish oil capsules taken daily for three months resulted in a decrease in anger levels that was not apparent in those taking the vegetable oil placebo. The results, published as a research abstract in the journal *Neuropsychopharmacology* (2006), indicate that fish oil has general mood-stabilizing properties. Following this, in March 2006, researchers from the University of Pittsburgh showed that among 106 healthy adults, those with the lowest blood levels of omega-3 were most likely to report mild depressive symptoms, a more negative outlook on life, and to be more impulsive.

Social sensitivity is a personality trait that refers to an individual's responsiveness to the perception of other people's judgments and reactions. Researchers from Wake Forest University reported recently that higher social sensitivity scores are associated with worse quality-of-life measurements among acne patients and are detrimental to social functioning. These findings have relevance to nutritional medicine because omega-3 fatty acids, and EPA in particular, have been shown to influence personality disorders. Omega-3 fatty acids are much lower in those with the extreme form of social sensitivity, social anxiety disorder. A study in *European Neuropsychopharmacology* (2006) showed that the blood levels of omega-3 fatty acids are well over 30 percent lower in those with social anxiety disorder. After determining that omega-3 fatty acids can cool anger in adults, Dr. Laure Buydens and colleagues from the New York Harbor Healthcare System showed in 2006 that fish oil rich in eicosapentaenoic acid can decrease anxiety in those with addiction disorders. Harvard researchers had previously shown in a 2003 placebo-controlled study that 1 gram of EPA significantly improves the symptoms of aggression and depression that characterize borderline personality disorder. These findings underscore the influence of omega-3 fatty acids on the development of various aspects of personality and behavior. They suggest that omega-3 fatty acids may alleviate and prevent some of the physiological and psychological aspects of acne.

Certain vitamins and minerals have also been found to be important in maintaining a balanced mood. Low blood levels of zinc, selenium, and folic acid have all been shown (individually) to be related to low mood states in humans. A common thread is that each of these nutrients helps to metabolize omega-3 fatty acids and boost omega-3 status. Patients with depression have blood-folate levels that are about 25 percent lower than adults without depression, and low blood levels of folate at baseline are predictive of a poor outcome with antidepressant therapies. Patients treated with Prozac who showed low blood-folate levels had a 42.9 percent relapse rate vs. only 3.2 percent relapse in those with the highest blood folate. In a large United Kingdom study, researchers placed half of adult subjects with depression on Prozac and 500 mcg of folic acid, and half on Prozac and a placebo. Significant improvements were noted in the Prozac and folic acid group—and fewer side effects from the medication were also reported in the folic acid group. For some reason, the logical third arm of this study, folic acid and a placebo, was never included. We suspect that folic acid itself, without the antidepressant medication, might have shown some benefit.

Looking at zinc, research shows that the blood zinc levels are between 12 and 16 percent lower among those with major depression, and indeed more severe depression correlates with lower zinc levels. The connection between low levels of zinc in depression and low levels of zinc in acne are almost certainly not coincidental. New clinical studies, the latest published in *Pharmacological Reports* (2005) show that just 25 mg of zinc daily can lead to significant improvement in depression and enhances the effectiveness of antidepressant medications. Isn't it interesting that three of the key ingredients in the antiacne prescription nutrient combo Nicomide include nutrients that have been tied to mediating human depression and anxiety—zinc, nicotinamide, and folic acid?

As mentioned, researchers from the Toyama Medical and Pharmaceutical University in Japan have been looking closely at the relationship between emotional stress and inflammation in acne. They have focused on the brain/nervous system chemical called substance P and stress-induced acne. Psychological stress can promote the release of substance P. In a paper published in the journal *Dermatology* (2003), the Japanese researchers reported that an abundance of nerves that release substance P surround and innervate the sebaceous glands of acne patients. Most researchers and clinicians consider substance P to be the pain signal; however, there is much more to this complex chemical. When released, substance P causes growth of the sebaceous gland and subsequent oil production to help fuel the acne bacterial growth and congestion in the follicle, and it also promotes inflammation. In addition, they reported that the enzymes responsible for clearing away substance P are controlled by zinc! In acne patients, this zinc-dependent enzyme that breaks down substance P and takes away its biological activity has been found to be unregulated and working overtime, setting the stage for a greater demand for zinc. When one considers that elevated levels of substance P in the brain may promote the symptoms of depression and anxiety, the plot certainly thickens.

As reported in *Nutritional Neuroscience* (2002), at least five studies have shown that low selenium levels are associated with a poor mood state—again, another interesting connection with the low selenium levels seen in acne. A 2003 study showed that selenium supplementation can curb anxiety in those with a high psychological burden. In addition, at least two controlled studies have also shown that a daily multivitamin can improve cognition and mood in otherwise healthy adults, particularly in those who have a poor background diet.

Another nutrient connected to depression and acne is worth noting—chromium. In a preliminary study published in *Medical Hypotheses* (1984), Dr. Mark McCarty of Pantox Laboratories reported improvements in acne with the administration of 400 micrograms of chromium per day. This is of interest for a few reasons, most notably that chromium has a well-deserved reputation as a regulator of blood-sugar levels, and that emerging studies are also showing antidepressant properties of chromium. So the mechanisms behind the benefits in acne might be due to its preventing insulin resistance and maintaining normal blood sugar. Recent placebo-controlled studies have also shown that chromium supplementation is helpful in alleviating depressive symptoms and carbohydrate cravings in depressed adults. Chromium is essential to life at minuscule concentrations, yet actually toxic at high concentrations and may cause cancer with chronically high exposure. Daily intake of chromium should not exceed 500 micrograms per day unless directed by a health-care professional. As with many nutrients, enough is wonderful, but too much is disastrous.

Finally, consideration should be given to vitamin B6, which has been shown to be helpful in premenstrual acne flare-ups. Interestingly, it is also involved in the metabolism of omega-3 fatty acids, and it, too, has been shown to be low in patients with depression. As reported in *Psychotherapy and Psychosomatics* (2004), low vitamin B6 levels are associated with severity of depression and may interfere with the normal manufacture of the mood-regulating brain chemical called serotonin.

Even dietary fiber intake has been connected to behavior, and—at its extreme end—suicide. In an enlightening study published in the journal *Nutrition* (2005), scientists compared detailed analyses of the diets of those who attempted suicide. Between a group of normal healthy adults and more than four hundred adults who had a lifetime history of suicide attempts, researchers found only two nutritional differences—the latter group had low polyunsaturated fat intake and low fiber intake. The polyunsaturated fat connection makes sense because these include the omega-3 fatty acids, well known to be involved in mood and behavior. But what about the fiber connection? How could low fiber possibly be connected to suicide? Dietary fiber is an indicator of more nutritious whole grains, fruits, and vegetables—foods that supply brain-critical vitamins, minerals, and antioxidant phytonutrients. Dietary fiber helps to reduce oxidative stress, and it promotes the growth of beneficial intestinal bacteria, which in turn may have direct and indirect effects on the central nervous system. It is also likely that dietary fiber decreases the production of the inflammatory immune chemicals that can disturb neurotransmission (nerve cell communication).

Dr. Andrew Smith and colleagues from Cardiff University, United Kingdom, found that a high-fiber (15 percent or more) breakfast cereal versus a low-fiber (3 percent) cereal seems to have a fatigue-reducing effect. Dr. Smith's study, published in the journal *Appetite* (2001), showed that a high-fiber breakfast is associated with less fatigue, less emotional distress, and fewer cognitive difficulties. The emotional distress connection is very interesting, because work from

Dr. Smith in *Nutritional Neuroscience* (2002) showed that regular consumption of quality breakfast cereal is associated with lower levels of the stress and acne-related hormone cortisol. Those with acne may want to forgo the milk and add a little cold Rice Dream; soymilk; or oat, almond (nut), or coconut milk to the fiber-rich cereal.

Fiber and Androgens

An additional area of consideration is the relationship between dietary fiber and androgens. There is no question that hormones, including the acne-causing androgens, can influence our moods and our behaviors. As previously discussed, there are now a number of studies that show the Western diet increases androgens (male hormones including testosterone). As long ago as 1979, researchers showed that switching from a traditional South African diet, high in fiber, to a typical North American low-fiber diet increased androgen levels. We also have the recent study by Dr. Christina Wang and colleagues from UCLA, which showed that reducing dietary fat and increasing dietary fiber lowered circulating androgen levels by 12 percent in healthy middle-aged men. The animal fat appears to be the issue rather than meat per se, because separate research using fatty meat, tofu, and lean meat showed that only *fatty* meat caused significant post-meal increases in testosterone.

Diet-induced elevations in androgens may also be fueling the anger in acne. When it comes to behavior, high testosterone has a well-established link to aggression in humans and animals. In a sample of almost forty-five hundred U.S. soldiers, higher testosterone levels were associated with job difficulties, antisocial behavior, marital difficulties, drug and alcohol abuse, and aggressive acts. Individuals with a background of aggressiveness, impulsive behaviors, and suicide attempts have higher levels of testosterone in the fluid that surrounds the central nervous system. In children, aggressiveness and antisocial behavior have been associated with higher testosterone and other androgens including dehydroepiandrosterone (DHEA). These are not massive differences in androgen levels. It is also likely that blood androgen levels are only a rough marker for total body androgen loads; even small relative increases appear to make a difference in behavior. Therefore, it is possible that dietary fiber can lower the risk of suicide by providing foods rich in nutrients, and also by modestly lowering the male hormone associated with suicide attempts.

Experimentally, chronic testosterone administration lowers levels of the so-called "feel good" brain chemical serotonin. The combination of low serotonin and elevated testosterone may set the stage for depression, aggression, anxiety, and anger. As we will discuss later, it is entirely possible that the changing Japanese diet is bringing with it changes in androgen levels, which in turn are influencing acne, the brain, and behavior.

In addition to protection against the oxidative stress of the acne process, research also suggests that antioxidants might influence mood and energy levels. Dietary antioxidants are also important to help preserve omega-3 fatty acids and prevent free-radical damage to the lipid components within nerve cells. Dietary antioxidants might not only prevent long-term cognitive decline later in life, but they may also influence mental state and mood in day-to-day life at younger ages as well. Support for this hypothesis comes from a University of Toronto study that showed consumption of a commercially available green food supplement (greens+, a powdered blend of twenty-three plant-based ingredients) increased energy and vitality when taken for three months versus a placebo. Green food supplements are known to be rich in antioxidants. As mentioned previously, antioxidants work together, much like an orchestra, with research showing that two antioxidants together have greater antioxidant potential than the sum of the two individual parts. While early research has shown vitamins A and C to be helpful in acne, they would probably be even more effective when taken with antioxidant-rich whole foods.

The availability of whole fruit, vegetable, and herbal extracts as powder is an exciting development in the supplement world. Modern extraction techniques can remove the water from fruits, vegetables, and herbs while leaving the nutrients behind. The powdered supplements in this category are generally referred to as "green food" supplements. They have been popular in Japan for decades. The first successful green food product introduced in North America was that by Canadian nutrition researcher Sam Graci. Author of *The Path to Phenomenal Health* (Wiley, 2005), he certainly did his homework when

THE BRAIN-SKIN CONNECTION

he put together his original and much-copied green food supplement more than ten years ago. The product in question, greens+, was recently the subject of two clinical studies.

The first study, published in the *Canadian Journal of Dietetic Practice and Research* (2004), involved more than a hundred otherwise healthy women from Toronto, Canada. They were instructed to take either greens+ or a carefully matched (placebo) powdered beverage for three months. Subjects were evaluated using various validated questionnaires. Those taking the actual greens+ were found to have improvements in vitality and had significantly more energy than those in the placebo group.

In a separate study, University of Toronto researchers found that greens+ does indeed increase blood antioxidant levels, and it lowers oxidative stress in otherwise healthy adults. According to the report by Dr. Venket Rao and his team from Toronto, the beneficial phytonutrients (polyphenols) in greens+ are well absorbed. This is important research because some scientists have questioned the absorption of antioxidants from whole foods and powdered formulas in humans. A food or extract can have a huge antioxidant activity when examined in a test tube, but if it isn't getting absorbed from the intestinal tract and into the bloodstream, then it really doesn't mean a whole lot.

It is our contention that this assumption that psychological dysfunction in acne is merely a result of the illness itself should be reevaluated. Too many similarities exist between nutritional influences

---

Genuine Health is the Toronto-based company that manufactures greens+, the supplement shown to improve energy levels among healthy but tired women in a University of Toronto–controlled study. This company has also combined a number of the antiacne nutrients we have highlighted (including EPA, zinc, and others) into a product called Perfect Skin. The supplement is commercially available in Canada, and at the time of writing it is the subject of a research trial in California. Each capsule contains 250 mg EPA derived from sardines, mackerel, and anchovies; 50 mg EGCG from green tea; 3.75 mg elemental zinc; 50 mcg selenium; 50 mcg chromium; and 2.5 mg vitamin E. See the appendix for more information about Perfect Skin.

on mental health and similar nutritional inadequacies in acne. As high-lighted in a study in the *British Journal of Dermatology* (1999), even with marked improvement using standard acne drugs, many patients have persisting emotional problems. The young teens and adults with low omega-3 levels and low zinc, selenium, chromium, and vitamin B6 lev-els are likely to be at higher risk of *both* acne and emotional disorders. There have been some hints in medical literature that acne patients have higher rates of emotional sensitivity before the onset of acne. Two small studies out of Germany and another from the British psychiatrist Dr. Eric Wittkower suggest that acne patients may already have higher levels of nervousness, anxiety, obsessions, and other emotional charac-teristics as part of their personality structure. The good news is, the very nutrients that might improve acne are the same nutrients shown to improve mood and decrease anger.

Stress and Acne Flare-Ups

Stress can be defined as the thoughts, feeling, behaviors, and phys-iological changes that occur when the demands placed upon you exceed your perceived ability to cope. The stress-related thoughts, feelings, behaviors, and physical changes are ultimately influenced by demands and perceptions. The average North American expe-riences about fifty brief stress response episodes per day! The stress "response" refers to the automatic physiological changes and accompanying thoughts that occur in the event of a perceived threat to our safety. It doesn't have to be a major trauma or life-altering stressor; even those daily hassles or minor annoyances are more than enough to trigger measurable elevations in blood levels of stress hormones from the adrenal gland—including the ones linked to acne, cortisol, and DHEA. Perceiving some amount of stress is a good thing; it allows us to adapt to changes and perform at our best. However, health problems arise when demands start to exceed our perceived ability to cope. Both chronic, daily hassles and major acute psychological trauma are well documented to compromise health.

For many years dermatologists have noted, at least clinically, that stress promotes acne flare-ups. As the rates of acne increase in adults, many experts are pointing a finger at stress as a causative player. It is interesting that many of the potentially antiacne nutrients are also known to lower the stress response. Take, for example, fish oil—it has been shown in a number of studies to lower stress hormones. In one study in the journal *Diabetes & Metabolism* (2003), three weeks of fish oil supplementation in the diets of healthy adult volunteers lowered the levels of the stress hormones epinephrine and cortisol after an experimental mental stress. As previously mentioned, levels of the primary stress hormone cortisol have been documented to be higher in both male and female acne patients. Magnesium, an important mineral that can dampen inflammation and decrease the release of sebum-stimulating substance P, lowers blood levels of the stress hormone cortisol under stressful circumstances in humans. On the other hand, chronic emotional stress is known to lower levels of magnesium in humans.

Numerous studies show that psychological stress increases oxidative stress, free-radical production, and low-grade inflammation, and causes a marked decline in the efficiency of the antioxidant defense system. In addition to lowering magnesium, acute and chronic mental stress is also associated with lower blood levels of two other potentially valuable antiacne minerals—zinc and selenium. Stress appears to lead to greater demand for the very minerals that may help keep acne in check.

The first formal research into the area of stress and acne was published in the *Journal of Laboratory and Clinical Medicine* (1953) when Dr. Thomas Lorenz and colleagues looked at the effects of inducing anger in experimental circumstances. These researchers found that a stressful interview, set up to purposely induce anger among the acne patients (males and females ages fifteen to thirty-one), caused an acne flare-up within a few days. Twenty-two of the subjects also kept a daily diary to document day-to-day emotional reactions to life experiences over extended periods. Once again there was a relationship between flare-ups in acne and emotional reactions including anger and remorse. In a review in *Medical Times* (1965) dermatologist William Kaufman of the Roanoke Memorial Hospital in Virginia stated that his clinical observations suggested that the competitive and emotional stress, "so characteristic of the social and scholastic competition in the acne-age group, are major causal factors."

In following the recurrent theme, lack of follow-up also applied to this area of acne research until Harvard Medical School dermatologist Robert Griesemer reported in 1978 that more than half of acne patients may have a worsening of symptoms in the days following emotional stress. The aggravation was typically noted about two days after the emotionally stressful episode. Then, in the *British Journal of Dermatology* (1997), Dr. C. I. Harrington from the Royal Hallamshire Hospital reported thirteen cases of adult acne in females, all of whom had clear complexions prior to the breakup of their marriages. Standard medications did little for the patients, while marked improvement in acne was noted after treatment with the antidepressant medication Prozac. Interestingly, almost three decades earlier, French researchers noted in *Marseille Medical* (1969) that a heart medication with antianxiety properties (propranolol) was very helpful in reducing sebum buildup and improving acne in adult patients. Even in women, stress is known to influence testosterone levels. For example, in women with anxiety, levels of testosterone are higher, while on the other hand, women with excellent stress-coping skills are protected against elevations in testosterone. Although large controlled studies are lacking, it is entirely plausible that treating the symptoms of depression and anxiety may lead to significantly improved complexion—particularly in those with stress-induced acne.

The acne-stress connection may influence acne particularly in females. Dermatologist Adam Reich and colleagues reported in *Dermatology Nursing* (2007) that even in young teens, females are five times more likely to indicate stress as an acne promoter. The increased rates of adult acne have been reported to be particularly high among professional women with high-stress jobs. This is interesting when considering that the stress hormone cortisol has been shown to be elevated in adults with acne. The effects of cortisol on the production of sebum have been documented since the early 1970s. As reported in the *Journal of Investigative Dermatology* (1974), there may be gender-specific effects of cortisol when it comes to sebum production. For reasons that are not entirely clear, females are much more sensitive to the effects of cortisol in sebum production than are males.

There are also differences in how stress, particularly work stress, might influence cortisol in the genders. Dr. Nanna Eller and colleagues from Denmark reported in *Biological Psychiatry* (2006) that cortisol is higher in women who work overtime, or take work home from the office. Furthermore, working women also have higher levels of cortisol on workdays, even higher than men, yet the cortisol levels of both genders are indistinguishable on days off! Cortisol levels are also associated with greater work demands, particularly if an individual is not in the upper economic brackets. Overall in women, increased time pressure, working hours, and subjective workload are associated with higher cortisol levels. This is not to say that cortisol is directly caus-

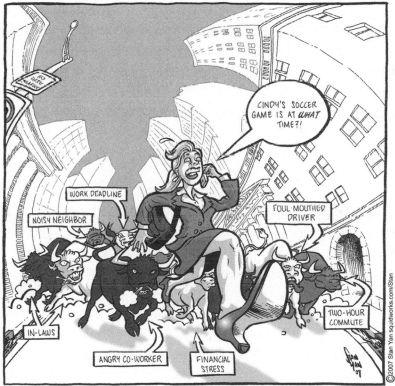

RUNNING OF THE BULLS.

ing acne; it is, however, a good marker to reflect other physiological changes brought on by stress—including inflammatory chemicals— changes that certainly appear to promote acne.

Dr. Lorena Arranz and colleagues reported in the *Journal of Psychosomatic Research* (2007) that women who were described as "anxious" had increased levels of cortisol, increased inflammatory immune chemicals, and diminished markers of antioxidant protection. Sadly, women who report high job stress are less likely to perform intentional leisure time exercise which has been shown to alleviate stress and anxiety. A study published in the *Scandinavian Journal of Medicine & Science in Sports* (2002) showed that physically active women experience better mental health, less depression, and better general health status. Of note, even low levels of intentional exercise, just one to two times per week, were positively correlated to women's mental health.

Another difference influencing the stress-acne connection in the genders may have to do with the effect of stress on testosterone and DHEA production via the adrenal glands. For men, some stress promotes testosterone production, while too much chronic stress causes a "threshold" and then a decline in testosterone levels. In contrast, Dr. Jean King and colleagues from the University of Massachusetts reported in *Neuroendocrinology Letters* (2005) that in women the "threshold" factor doesn't come into play. If you keep piling on the stress in women, the testosterone keeps going up in a direct and linear fashion. This direct influence of androgens may be further fueling acne in women under chronic stress.

The stress-acne connection has had its detractors. Remember that Australian study where the researchers queried medical students on the eve of graduation about acne and diet? Well, in the same study the authors were also shocked to find that 67 percent of the soon-to-be MDs strongly believed in a stress-acne connection. This figure is not too far off the 74 percent of patients actually with acne who firmly believed that stress and anxiety can exacerbate the condition. Here again these researchers blame the community of laypeople for this so-called "misconception," writing in the *Australasian Journal of Dermatology* (2001) they stated, "In particular stress, diet, lifestyle and personal hygiene are often erroneously claimed to be important factors."

Just two years later the relationship between stress and acne would be given a solid dose of credibility with the publication of a study by Stanford University medical student (and now doctor) Annie Chiu and colleagues. The investigators looked at the influence of exam stress on the severity of acne among a diverse group of male and female university students. Dermatologist Alexa Kimball graded the subjects' acne severity using validated techniques and without knowledge of the students' perceived stress scores. An additional dermatologist was required to provide independent verification of acne severity using digital photographs. The results, published in the *Archives of Dermatology* (2003), showed very clearly that students who reported the greatest increases in perceived stress during examination periods also displayed the greatest exacerbation of acne severity—and the relationship between stress and acne occurred in a very linear and predictable manner. More stress translated into greater acne. That is not all; in the study, the researchers also queried the students on dietary habits before and during the stressful exam periods. They asked the students to rate dietary quality on a scale from poor to excellent, and wouldn't you know it, the students who reported a worsening of dietary quality also had increased acne severity! This connection between stress, acne, and self-reports of a drop in dietary quality should not be entirely surprising because there is an abundance of research on stress-induced alterations to a healthy diet.

Both acute and chronic stressors have the potential to negatively influence our food choices, which in turn can promote acne and its severity. While research shows that not everyone alters their eating habits under stress, the vast majority, more than 80 percent of us, do

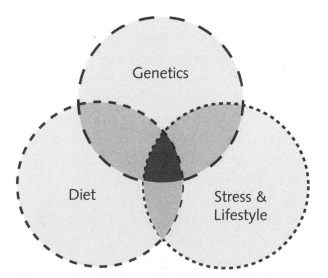

The Acne Triad—Genetics influence lifetime acne risk, diet and stress influence each other, and both influence genetic expression.

make changes. For some, the change may be a drastic reduction in food intake, while for others it may be a significant elevation in caloric intake via foods high in sugar and saturated fat. Whatever dietary direction in which stress may take an individual, it is the high-quality, nutrient-dense foods that are abandoned. More than 70 percent of those who both undereat and overeat during stress report an increase in snacking on foods that can hardly be described as nutritional powerhouses. The fats and sugars provide a very brief palatable comfort and then go on to spike insulin, gum up the follicle, and promote inflammation.

In a study published in the journal *Psychosomatic Medicine* (1990), researchers from the University of Washington showed that employees changed their dietary habits at times of major work deadlines. Dietary intake of total calories, total fat, and the percentage of calories from fat were significantly higher in periods before deadlines than in more quiescent periods. Any dietary plan, be it to lose weight or improve brain health, that ignores such research is clearly incomplete. Around the same time, French researchers reported that total caloric intake among high school students increased during stressful exam periods versus subsequent nonexamination days. This, of course, is in line with the newer research from Stanford University that connected stressful exam periods, poor dietary habits, and acne flare-ups.

Dr. Andrew Steptoe of the University of London and his colleagues reported in the *British Journal of Health Psychology* (1998) that annoying minor daily stressors and hassles can trigger unhealthy eating habits. Among the nurses and teachers enrolled in the study, there was a significant (37 percent) increase in fast-food consumption during high-stress periods. Men in particular turned to eating beef, lamb, and pork with a 45 percent increase during times of stress. The research also supported the notion that cheese and sweet foods are indeed comfort (or mood-driven) foods. In a more recent 2003 study in *Health Psychology*, researchers found that among more than four thousand teens, greater self-reported stress levels were tightly correlated with more fatty food intake and less fruit and vegetable consumption. In addition, the adolescents who reported greater stress were more likely to consume nutrient-poor snacks.

In a study presented at the North American Association for the

Study of Obesity's Annual Scientific Meeting in Vancouver (2005), researchers from the University of Kansas showed that at the end of a six-month weight-loss regimen, those who reported the highest levels of stress and depression were more likely to regain weight. Self-reported stress and depressive symptoms were associated with greater amounts of fat and total calories consumed when assessed at various points from nine to eighteen months later. These results add to the evidence that stress can influence unhealthy dietary choices and compromise the ability to maintain a lean body and, quite likely, a clear complexion.

Interestingly, those who have the highest blood levels of the stress hormone cortisol in reaction to experimental stress are particularly prone to eating the wrong types of foods, especially those high in sugar and fat. The most recent study, published in *Psychoneuro-endocrinology* (2007), showed that when adults were challenged with an experimental stressor, certain individuals responded with very high cortisol levels. Upon further review, these were the subjects who were most likely to resort to snacking in association with the stress of daily hassles.

Overactivity of the stress branch of the nervous system, the sympathetic branch, is associated with overeating, changes in blood hormones, and a decrease in the amino acid called tryptophan. Overactivity of the sympathetic branch, also called an increase in "sympathetic tone," impairs digestion and interferes with sleep. We know from the previous chapter that chronic stress and impaired digestion have the potential to impact our beneficial intestinal bacteria and, by extension, our inflammation-oxidative stress load. However, lower tryptophan availability is a really big deal because it is a building block for the mood-regulating neurotransmitter called serotonin. Low levels of serotonin are, in turn, associated with depressed mood, insomnia, anxiety, anger, and the further consumption of sugary and calorie-dense carbohydrates. Remember that most antidepressant medications influence serotonin levels in the brain. Researchers from Innsbruck Medical University in Austria have performed research in the area of inflammation and tryptophan availability. They have found that inflammatory chemicals, even at low levels, are capable of breaking down tryptophan. The same group recently showed that

Saint-John's-wort (SJW) can prevent tryptophan breakdown in the presence of inflammation, so this may be an important mechanism behind the SJW action as a natural antidepressant. One mechanism whereby stress- and acne-promoting inflammatory chemicals and cytokines can alter mood and sleep is through changing tryptophan availability. We reviewed the relationships between fish consumption and protection against acne and stress. Beyond the fish oil and omega-3 story, it is also important to note that fish boosts blood tryptophan levels much more than comparative meals of chicken or beef. Writing in the *Journal of Nutrition* (1992), Australian researchers speculated that not only were the blood tryptophan levels higher after consuming fish (versus similar portions of chicken or beef), there was also a greater sense of satiety (fullness) after eating fish. The researchers speculated that more blood tryptophan translates into more brain serotonin levels, hence the feeling of satiety. So at this point we think it's fair to say that fish is a true antistress food with multiple health benefits.

Green tea is arguably the ultimate antistress beverage, and given the stress-acne connections and the higher levels of the stress hormone cortisol that have been documented in acne, green tea should not be overlooked. Researchers from the University of Montpellier in France recently reported in *Brain Research* (2006) that EGCG within green tea can lower the stress response by its actions on the GABA system in the brain. GABA (gamma-amino benzoic acid) is the major inhibitory brain chemical, inhibitory because it is largely responsible for checking the system and preventing overload. For example, those prone to panic attacks have low levels of GABA in certain parts of the brain, and GABA dysfunction has been implicated in other anxiety disorders, mood disorders and attention deficit/hyperactivity disorder. Under stressful conditions, GABA levels are depleted. Recently, a team of researchers from Kyoto Women's University reported in *Biofactors* (2006) that 100 mg of naturally fermented GABA induced relaxation and reduced anxiety in healthy young adults. Furthermore, under stressful conditions, volunteers with a history of phobic-anxiety in the GABA group had a more beneficial immune-system profile and did not experience the immune-system depression typical of anxiety and stress.

Green tea is also particularly rich in an amino acid called L-theanine, and since theanine stimulates GABA production as well as the feel-good neurotransmitter serotonin, this may be the reason for the lack of jitteriness after consuming green tea versus an energy drink or a coffee. As highlighted by Dr. Kenta Kimura in the journal *Biological Psychology* (2007), emerging research shows that theanine promotes mental functioning yet also has antistress properties that calm the brain. Theanine levels are much lower in black tea and in green teas grown in nonshaded areas. The levels are highest in matcha green tea, which is grown in shaded areas within certain locales in Japan. With all the potential benefits, it is no wonder that many people claim that drinking green tea has made a significant difference in their acne.

Cutting off the Stress-Acne Cycle

The mechanisms behind stress-induced acne probably involve numerous pathways. For starters, stress can increase the production of androgens, those "male" hormones known to be involved in the acne process. Stress is most likely to promote androgen production when it is viewed as competitive stress. In other words, jockeying for position in heavy traffic, working extra hours to keep up with the work-based competition/promotions and just generally spinning the wheels of the modern-day commercial rat race is more than enough to influence androgen levels. Have you ever noticed how people can "change" personalities when there are competitive stakes to the outcome? In many ways our society has now become one big competition. Even the anticipation of competition has been shown to influence androgen levels. This means that merely getting ready to negotiate a crowded mall in anticipation of fighting for the hot new video game (or whatever the consumer item du jour might be) is enough to get the acne-promoting androgens flowing in both men and women.

Stress may influence the enhanced production of the nervous system chemical called Substance P, and prolonged stress, at least experimentally, causes growth in the number of substance P nerve fibers that innervate the skin. Substance P release in turn can promote anxiety when at work in the brain and promote acne worsening sebum production when working at the sebaceous gland. As highlighted by

Does Coffee Promote Acne?

Coffee has been unfairly vilified and associated with most chronic health conditions, and acne is no exception. As stated in a review in *Harvard Women's Health Watch* (2004): "The latest research discounts the notion that moderate coffee consumption—which we interpret to be about 2–4 cups per day—causes significant or lasting harm. Indeed, some studies suggest that coffee and caffeine may offer some real health benefits." Despite the suggestions by some Internet sources, there is no evidence that coffee aggravates acne.

Research shows that on a per-serving basis, coffee is in the top five highest sources of antioxidants for North Americans, along with blackberries, walnuts, strawberries, artichokes and cranberries. Coffee is particularly effective at protecting lipids (fats) against oxidative stress which may have relevance in acne. It is often stated that coffee promotes a stress response, although in reality this may be apparent only in those who do not drink coffee on a regular basis. In fact, a new study in *FEBS Letters* (2006) shows that the constituents of coffee (not caffeine) can dampen the activity of the enzyme (11β-HSD) responsible for producing active cortisol. This might help explain why a number of studies have shown that both caffeinated and decaf coffee consumption correlate with improved glucose tolerance, insulin sensitivity, and reduced risk of type 2 diabetes.

We find it telling that in the Iowa Women's Health Study (evaluating more than twenty-seven thousand women for fifteen years), the consumption of one to three cups of coffee per day was associated with a 24 percent reduction in the risk of cardiovascular death and a 33 percent reduction in the risk of dying from any condition rooted in inflammation.

Coffee is obviously not for everyone, and it may cause anxiety and insomnia in sensitive individuals. It is also important to note that the "cups" we refer to are traditional home-brewed cups, not to be confused with those used in commercial chains with Italian-sounding sizes—these can have more than five times the caffeine content per "cup." We also caution against the popular milk shakes that disguise themselves as "coffee"; some of them contain in excess of 500 calories and 27 grams of fat.

Dr. Karl Ebner of Innsbruck University in the journal *Amino Acids* (2006), anti–substance P medications have recently been shown to have significant antianxiety properties. Stress also causes an increase in the production of those inflammatory immune chemicals called cytokines, which, in turn, can influence free-radical production and oxidative stress.

Psychosocial stressors can also promote the production of the acne-inducing hormone IGF-1. Interestingly, researchers have shown that IGF-1 levels are high in depression and decrease with remission. As reported in *Psychoneuroendocrinology* (2000), when antidepressant medications are abruptly discontinued, there are significant increases in blood IGF-1 levels in conjunction with symptoms. Research published in the *International Journal of Environmental Health* (2004) suggested that airborne environmental pollutants from traffic congestion and psychosocial stressors may work in tandem to elevate IGF-1 levels in stress-prone humans.

Stressors, as discussed, also cause us to choose the very foods we should avoid—foods high in sugar and high in fat (animal and vegetable oils). This spikes blood sugar, enhances sebum production, and promotes inflammation. Of course, when we are overconsuming calorie-dense and nutritionally poor foods, we are also shunning the nutrient-rich foods we desperately need. Acute and chronic stressors lead to great demands for magnesium, zinc, and selenium, and without dietary replenishment the flames of inflammation and oxidative stress burn more intensely. When acute stress turns chronic, an entire cascade of hormones, inflammatory chemicals, and free radicals left unchecked can lead to fertile ground for acne.

The good news is that just as there is the "fight-or-flight" response to stress, with its cascade of damaging stress hormones, inflammatory chemicals, and free radicals, so, too, is there an innate mirror image to the stress response—it is called the relaxation response. This physiological process promotes healing, rest, and digestion. The calming branch of the nervous system, the parasympathetic branch, becomes dominant when the relaxation response becomes dominant. In chapter 8, "Action Plan for the Clear Skin Diet," we will discuss the relaxation response in greater detail as part of your plan to promote clear skin.

If we can confidently predict that mental stressors promote acne, we should also expect the interventions that help us appropriately manage stress and induce the relaxation response to be helpful in reducing acne. Incredibly, this area of research is mostly barren. Despite a wealth of research that demonstrates the value of psychological interventions and the induction of the relaxation response in a wide variety of stress-related conditions, acne has been left untouched. Well . . . almost. We do have one study to draw from, an interesting evaluation of the effects of mental imagery and biofeedback relaxation on acne treatment outcome.

There are many types of biofeedback, a mind-body medicine modality in which we can learn conscious control over physiological processes. In this case, the acne patients used EMG biofeedback, in which they learned muscular relaxation through observations with a machine that measured electrical activity of the muscles. The cognitive imagery technique involved the acne patients' using mental images that might be associated with the healing process. For example, one patient used the imagery of a farmer digging out the clogged follicles and then cleansing the channel of the pore with a bucket of liquid medication. Another patient visualized the opening of the follicles wider and wider with the depth of the muscular relaxation to allow the oil and bacteria to flow out. Both EMG biofeedback and mental imagery have been used successfully to improve the outcomes of many stress-related conditions. The results were positive, and as reported in the *Journal of Psychosomatic Research* (1983), the twelve sessions significantly reduced acne severity and enhanced the effectiveness of standard acne care among those in the biofeedback-imagery group. Interestingly, the last line written in their publication was, "The necessary and sufficient components of the relaxation-imagery treatment should be identified via future research." That was almost twenty-five years ago, and, despite the justification, we are still waiting for more research using psychological interventions in acne.

Remember that stress increases hormones that create the "fight-or-flight" reaction. That is, your body is preparing to defend itself against a perceived threat of harm by either fighting the enemy or fleeing from it. The hormones prepare your body, as noted stress expert Dr. Robert Sapolsky says, "for a sudden explosion of muscular activity." With this in mind, an excellent stress-busting technique is exercise; muscular activity is what your body is often calling out for in the stressful setting. Research reviews have concluded that moderate regular exercise should be considered a viable means of treating depression and anxiety disorders, and improving mental well-being for all. Research shows that exercise enhances the production of a brain chemical called neuropeptide Y. Low levels of neuropeptide Y are associated with depressive symptoms, and higher levels are associated with resilience to stress—certainly something to consider in the acne-stress connection.

Chapter 8 will provide specific guidance on exercise and the relaxation response. However, it is also worthwhile to highlight some of the general themes of stress management and the influence of mind over healing at this point—we will later address techniques and considerations that reinforce the relaxation response and exercise plan.

Lesson from the Placebo

The idea that mind and body are separate and distinct from each other has lingered around the medical profession for centuries. This separatist notion has finally been put to rest in recent years with the volumes of research on how humans respond to placebos used in clinical studies. The placebo is nothing more than an inert, look-alike pill without active physiological components—it is also referred to as a sugar pill. Despite the absence of medicinal ingredients, more than 35 percent of subjects in clinical trials respond to the placebo. The placebo response in stress-related emotional and digestive disorders can reach almost 80 percent. In acne it has been documented to be as high as 56 percent. Clearly, individuals who have a *belief* that they are taking a chemically active pill or herb can influence their own illness progression. Recent studies have documented physiological changes, even in the brain itself, among those who believe they are taking a medication (actually a placebo). Consider that the placebo effect in acne is quite high, in some cases as high as 56 percent. In other words, acne patients who have received nothing more than a sugar pill have been documented to have a 50 percent reduction in the severity of acne—this speaks volumes to the power of belief and psychological influences on the course of acne.

The lesson of the placebo tells us that there is a significant effect of the mind on the course of illness. To promote optimal health, and a clear complexion, the goal is to grab the thought processes and lessons of the placebo effect and utilize them, make them work for you in health promotion—this is where mind-body medicine comes in. The discipline involves techniques and therapies that take into full consideration that the mind (thoughts and emotions) can influence behavior and health status. Mind-body medicine also considers the influence of a disordered body on thoughts and emotions. The techniques of mind-body medicine include, but are not limited to, meditation, hypnotherapy, biofeedback, guided imagery and visualization, yoga, prayer, tai chi, breathing exercises, therapeutic writing, and art, music, and dance, and perhaps most important, cognitive-behavioral therapy. There are more than two thousand studies in well-respected medical journals that give credibility to the value of mind-body medicine.

Meditation

The practice of meditation can be traced back more than three thousand years to the Indian subcontinent. There are two main categories of meditation—mindfulness and concentration. The focus of mindfulness meditation is to stay in the "here and now." Through practice, one learns to pay attention to what one is experiencing in the current moment, without drifting off to worry of the future or experiences of the past. Mindfulness involves suspending judgment and letting go of opinions, thus becoming less reactive, and of importance to acne, less angry. This fosters acceptance, self-reflection, and greater ability to handle difficulties without avoidance.

Mindfulness has been the subject of much scientific inquiry, and recent studies highlight its value in stress management. In a study in the *Journal of Personality and Social Psychology* (2003), researchers showed that greater awareness and being mindful in life from day to day are correlated with enhanced well-being. Among the fifteen hundred adults surveyed, higher scores on a scale of mindfulness were associated with improved mood, optimism, life satisfaction, and willingness to attempt new experiences. Individuals were assessed on mindfulness using fifteen questions, including those related to mental focus in the present and preoccupation with past and future—one question in particular was directly related to a mindfulness-diet connection: "Do you snack without being aware that you are eating?" Answering yes to this question may be a sign you should work on mindfulness. Another example of the need for mindfulness would be forgetting someone's name two seconds after they have told you.

Mindfulness meditation is a very portable technique—it can be conducted while seated and enhanced with meditative breathing; it can also work well with yoga or while walking in a slow and observant fashion. Meditative breathing is otherwise known as diaphragmatic breathing where it is the abdomen, and not the upper chest, that moves in and out. Some suggest placing your hand over your belly button, feel it move with your breaths, and imagine a balloon being inflated. You can think of the air flow in abdominal breathing as "in and down" as you develop a natural abdominal movement.

Concentration meditation removes focus from the everyday hassles, worries, aggravations, and all that makes our minds cluttered and stressed. The focus, instead, is an object (e.g., a picture or a candle), a word/phrase/mantra, or a visualized object. Perhaps the best-known form of concentration meditation is the *relaxation response* developed by Dr. Herbert Benson of Harvard Medical School and the world-renowned Mind-Body Medical Institute. After scientifically evaluating the physiological effects of Transcendental Meditation, Dr. Benson came to learn that focusing attention on a simple mental stimulus (word, phrase, image) in conjunction with relaxed breathing brought about a reduction in sympathetic (stress branch) nervous system activity, lower heart rate, decreased muscle tension, lower blood pressure, and a respiratory rate in the completely opposite direction from anxiety-related hyperventilation. What he found was that, just as there is a well-defined and automatic stress response, so, too, there is an opposing relaxation response that can be brought on by a form of meditation.

Music Therapy

Music has been used for centuries as a means to enhance mood and well-being. Researchers from Case Western Reserve University and the Tzu-Chi General Hospital in Taiwan showed that sedative music selections, listened to for forty-five minutes at bedtime, improved sleep duration and quality. There was also less daytime sleepiness and improved mental functioning. Relaxing music has also been shown to prevent sharp rises in cortisol after psychological stressors.

Yoga/Tai Chi

Yoga and tai chi are mind-body medical interventions that bring together physical movement and emotional being. Recent studies have documented the stress-lowering values of both these modalities. Hatha (physical) is a popular form of yoga that incorporates specific movements and postures (asana), as well as breathing techniques (pranayama) which are often used along with meditation. Yoga has been shown to improve sleep and reduce the perception of stress. Since anger might be involved in worsening the course of acne, it is of note that a number of studies show yoga can lower anger levels. Research published in the *Annals of Behavioral Medicine* (2004) showed that yoga can reduce cortisol levels and improve scores on the Perceived Stress Scale. Tai chi also combines physical movement, breathing, and meditation. The coordinated breathing and movement are said to enhance the flow of energy (*qi*, pronounced chee) throughout the body. As with yoga, tai chi has also been shown to reduce the stress hormone cortisol.

See Green

As previously discussed, there is some published research that indicates rural dwellers are at decreased risk of acne. This may be related to an increased likelihood that those in rural regions are more likely to hold on to healthy, traditional eating habits. The decreased risk also may be related to lowered levels of stress outside concrete jungles. The urban environment can bring with it more daily hassles, noise, substance misuse, insufficient light, tight living quarters, and, despite millions of people, social isolation. A number of published studies have suggested that the urban environment is a risk factor for emotional disorders. For example, a large study in the *British Journal of Psychiatry* (2004) showed that those in urban environments are up to 20 percent more likely to experience depression than rural dwellers.

One factor related to the urban environment is the presence of concrete, bricks, steel, and tar along with the relative absence of greenery when compared to rural environments. Writing in the *American Journal of Public Health* (2004), Drs. Frances Kuo and Andrea Taylor of the University of Illinois found that outdoor activities conducted in green (natural) settings improved attention and reduced hyperactivity more than the same activities conducted in built outdoor (urban-style) and indoor settings. The age, gender, income, community type, or geographic region made no difference—only that the activity be conducted in a green, natural environment.

As proposed by environmental psychologist Dr. Stephen Kaplan, the reason we feel so refreshed after time spent in natural settings is that in nature there is little effort required to inhibit or suppress unwanted stimuli. In unnatural settings such as sitting in front of a computer screen in an office, or shopping in a crowded, colorful mall, there is a requirement to deliberately direct attention to the task at hand, and to actively avoid a multitude of unwanted stimuli. All of this promotes stress, while seeing green appears to ground us from overload. Dr. Kuo and her colleagues, as well as other researchers, have shown that nature-based environments can lower stress, improve cognition, and reduce impulsive behavior.

Another reason to get outdoors and see some green, or even better, to put yourself in a forest environment, has to do with the exposure to negative ions and other natural chemicals that are absent in the air of urban environments. Days with high air pollution have been associated with a disproportionate number of mental health emergency calls. As mentioned in chapter 4, Hormones and the Clear Skin Diet, environmental pollutants in the typical urban setting can lead to significant elevations in the acne-generating IGF-1 levels. The influence of unnatural environmental chemicals on mood, perceived stress, concentration, and cognitive functioning has been documented over the years.

Negative air ions are natural components of air and breath that are depleted within polluted, enclosed, and air-conditioned rooms.

Negative ions are also lowered by electronic devices, such as computer screens and televisions found in homes and offices. Negative air ions are known to influence mood in a generally positive way, and are much higher in natural settings, after rain, near oceans, waterfalls and inside woodlands. According to research published in the journal *Indoor Air* (2004), negative air ions have been shown to promote our antioxidant defense system and improve blood flow. Small machines that generate negative air ions indoors are effective in treating seasonal affective disorder (SAD or the winter blues), and a recent study in the journal *Psychological Medicine* (2005) indicates that they can help lift mood in nonseasonal depression as well. Research published in the *International Journal of Biometeorology* (2005) shows that patients prone to panic attacks are much less likely to experience panic after rain when negative ion count is high.

In Japan, the practice of forest-air bathing is called *shinrin-yoku*, and it has been used medicinally for many years. In a study also published in the *International Journal of Biometeorology* (1998), researchers from the Hokkaido School of Medicine showed that walking in forest air lowers the stress hormone cortisol and improves well-being. The effects of woodland walking appear to enhance the value of exercise alone. The researchers suggest that at least some of the benefits are related to the volatile compounds within the forest air. Further support for forest walking comes from a study in *Public Health* (2007), where it was shown to lower hostility and depressive symptoms compared to exercise in other environments, and even compared to engaging in enjoyable recreational activities.

The Eating Environment

The dietary context, the environment in which we eat our meals and snacks, can have a profound influence on the overall calories consumed and the dietary quality. Research published in the *Journal of the American Dietetic Association* (2003) showed that high TV/video use was associated with increased consumption of soft drinks, fried foods, and snacks among four thousand adolescents. Greater weekday TV viewing was also associated with more frequent visits to fast-food establishments among teens, where typical consumption involves high-sugar, high-saturated/trans-fat foods and beverages.

It has also been shown that more weekly TV viewing goes hand in hand with a higher BMI and greater requests for commonly advertised foods. We're sure you can guess what kinds of foods are being marketed to young people on TV. Almost 80 percent of food advertised during those shows watched by youngsters is junk food, with sweets, candy and soft drinks accounting for 44 percent of the total. Researchers have found that food advertisements increase children's preferences for high-fat and high-carbohydrate foods. Belgian researchers showed that on the average, just one hour of TV watching equals the consumption of 156 calories. When you take away physical activity, 156 calories per hour of TV over time can really add to the waistline and compromise brain health.

According to a detailed review published in the *Journal of Adolescence* (2004), video games significantly increase stress. The sound tracks of violent video games include techno and heavy metal music, which adds to the stress response. Researchers from the University of Montreal showed that techno music significantly increases cortisol levels in video-game players versus silent conditions. Therefore, extended periods spent playing most video games increase chronic stress and cortisol, may increase the propensity to anger/violence, decrease physical activity, promote obesity, and overstimulate the system.

Relaxing Aromas

The beneficial effects of certain aromas on the human psyche have been documented for centuries. The human olfactory (smell) system is intricately tied to our emotional control center known as the limbic system. Even simply talking about an aroma can bring emotions and memories to the conscious level.

Essential oils are capable of reducing stress, promoting relaxation, and enhancing cognitive function—it all depends on the oil itself and personal preferences. Research on lavender, rosemary, and peppermint has shown them to improve mood and promote a sense of contentment. Researchers from Japan have also shown that lavender can help dampen down the sympathetic, or stress, branch of the nervous system.

Researchers from the Wheeling Jesuit University found that jasmine may promote sleep quality and increase alertness the following day. They examined the effects of jasmine, lavender, or no scent for three nights. The aromatherapy was infused into the rooms at such low levels that many were not even aware of any aroma at all. Not only did the jasmine sleepers toss and turn less frequently, they woke up feeling less anxiety the next day. The jasmine sleepers also performed better on cognitive testing the next day, and lavender also showed some benefit.

The same group from Wheeling recently showed that peppermint and cinnamon aromatherapy might quell the anger associated with road rage. They showed that prolonged driving led to the expected increased anger, fatigue, and physical demand, as well as decreased energy. Peppermint and cinnamon both decreased driving frustration and increased alertness while driving, and, interestingly, the aroma of fast food made things worse!

Sauna

Heat-based therapy has been used as a means to relax, cleanse, and purify the body for thousands of years. Anecdotal reports by some suggest that sauna use is helpful in acne because it "opens up the pores." In reality, sauna use may be helpful in acne for other reasons. Researchers from Kagoshima University in Japan have been examining the physiological influences of sauna as a medical therapy.

The Japanese researchers, led by Dr. Akinori Masuda, showed in 2004 that saunas lower blood pressure and oxidative stress. Therefore, in addition to being psychologically relaxing, we now know that they are reducing free radicals.

Writing/Journaling

Taking advantage of therapeutic writing involves expression of your deepest emotions, including what you feel and why you feel it. Research shows that confronting difficult life experiences through writing and art can have very positive effects on both emotional and physical well-being. There are more than a dozen studies that indicate writing about stressful or traumatic events can improve various health conditions. Write as if it is just for you, this way you will be less likely to hold back. If stressful events or the stress related to your complexion are constantly on your mind, it may be time to write things down or draw them out.

Stress-Hardiness

It may be helpful to try to learn from those individuals who seem to easily deflect stress. Dr. Suzanne Kobasa of the City University of New York identified three defining, and consistent, characteristics of so-called "stress-hardiness." These folks have been found to embrace the three Cs of daily life—Challenge, Control, and Commitment. Stress-resilient individuals see change as a challenge, something that is normal and to be viewed as a stimulus for growth and maturity rather than a threat. With regard to control, hardy personalities believe their actions do make a difference. They believe that they do have control and they are not merely victims of fate. While they may have no more control over events than those who are stress-prone, they simply believe they do. Finally, stress-hardy individuals are highly committed to what they pursue in life.

Additional Notes

Other general considerations include but are not limited to organizational skills, time management, prioritizing tasks and life goals, delegating, letting go of procrastination, using humor, being optimistic, taking advantage of social support, and getting proper sleep. It is also important to appreciate recreation and take time out for yourself. Step away from the computer and take some time for yourself—remember that computer screens and photocopy machines increase free-radical production (oxidative stress) in humans. New research shows that extended periods at visual-display terminals (monitors) cause mental fatigue and increase both oxidative and psychological stress.

Take a break, limit your computer use, and turn off your cell phone once in a while—research shows that mobile phones blur the boundaries between home and work, an important consideration for stressed working adults with acne. Research in the *Journal of Marriage and Family* (2005) showed that cell phone use is linked to heightened psychological distress and reduced family satisfaction. Cell phones cause work to spill over into the home.

Even in the absence of high-quality studies using stress-management techniques in acne, there is every reason to believe these techniques should be part and parcel of acne care. If stress promotes acne, which the research shows that it does, then lifestyle modifications that minimize stress should help. Finding the technique that works for you and fitting it into your life can be a challenge. In chapter 8, Action Plan for the Clear Skin Diet, we will concentrate on exercise and Dr. Herbert Benson's relaxation response. to give you concrete recommendations so you can make the changes that work for you.

Chapter Key Points

✔ Acne causes not only social and self-esteem issues, it is also associated with clinical depression.

✔ Many of the same nutrient insufficiencies that relate to depression are also tied to acne—omega-3 fatty acids, zinc, selenium, chromium, magnesium, fiber, vitamin A, and other antioxidants.

✔ Acne worsens in many people during times of stress.

✔ Stress can alter dietary practices—overall calorie, fat, and sugar intake increases while fruit and vegetable intake falls off.

✔ Competitive stress increases the acne hormones—androgens and IGF-1.

✔ Preliminary research suggests that inducing the innate relaxation response (opposite of the stress response) using biofeedback improves acne.

✔ While specific studies in acne have not yet confirmed the usefulness of activities that induce the relaxation response, research from other medical disciplines suggests value in treating many illnesses connected to stress.

✔ The Clear Skin Diet Action Plan will provide comprehensive catalog of ways to induce the relaxation response.

7

The Former Clear Skin Nation: Japan

A S WE HAVE DISCUSSED, THE diets and lifestyle of certain isolated ethnic communities are reported to provide great protection against acne. The dietary insulation against acne by traditional diets is derived from both inclusion and exclusion—that is, the high quality of the nutrients included in the diet, as well as the absence of non-nutritive, blood-sugar-spiking processed items and inflammation-promoting vegetable-oil/saturated-fat-laden foods. Although many of the particular foods consumed in these isolated communities are very unique and generally not available in North American markets, we can still draw from the basic dietary backgrounds. The unique diets of the Kitavan Islanders of Papua New Guinea, the Aché community of Paraguay, the Peruvian Indians in Arequipa, the Okinawan Islanders of Japan, and the Inuit living in polar regions all provide the common threads of . . .

1. Less processed foods

2. More colorful antioxidants

3. Greater intake of omega-3 fatty acids

4. Fewer foods capable of spiking blood sugar

5. More fiber

From a practical standpoint, however, it may be most worthwhile to look at the particulars of the traditional Japanese diet as *the* clear skin, antiacne diet. Keep in mind that just a few decades ago, the rates of acne in Japan were much lower than those in the United States, so obviously something has happened along the way since then.

Japanese dermatologists had been noting a rise in the incidence of acne that correlated with the dietary changes and affluence that followed the end of the war in 1945. Most of the population studies were published only in Japanese-language journals and were therefore not part of Western medical literature. Noted Japanese dermatologist Kasue Ohara provided rare insight into the rates and treatment of acne in Japan in a commentary published in the *Journal of the American Medical Women's Association* (1969). Although Dr. Ohara described similar conventional approaches as used in Western medicine (topical and oral medications), she also noted that a healthy low-fat, low-carbohydrate diet, adequate sleep, and the avoidance of psychological stressors were emphasized by Japanese dermatologists. Regarding acne, she stated that "statistical data reported in Japan show a tendency to a gradual increase in incidence. The incidence started several years after World War II, namely 1950, when the post-war era was over." These were minor changes, and they were the writing on the wall that bigger changes to the acne rates were yet to come. Despite the minor changes, Dr. Ohara referenced rates of acne through the 1960s which were still, on average, 50 percent lower than in North America. Recall that in 1964, Dr. Harumi Terada of the University of Tokyo, after conducting a large study, concluded that extensive acne was much more common among young Americans than in their counterparts living in Tokyo and Yokohama. Actually the rates of acne among the Japanese were about half that of age-matched Americans—numbers very similar to the population studies described by Dr. Ohara.

Here we are some forty years later, and the rates of acne are almost identical in Japan and North America. As you might imagine two nutritionally oriented doctors would do, we look to the environment, including diet and lifestyle factors that may explain such changes. Thanks to international record keeping on per-capita dietary quality within nations, we can go back in time to the 1960s and examine the major differences between the Japanese and North American diets.

The graphs that follow tell an interesting story about the changing Japanese diet, and they highlight some major differences among key dietary groups in North America and Japan. The much lower intakes of meat, milk, animal fats, sugars, white potatoes, and vegetable oils are all among the candidates that played a role in genetic influences on the expression of acne. In addition, the inclusion of anti-inflammatory, omega-3 fatty-acid-rich fish and seafood may have played a protective role in 1964. White potatoes, known to spike insulin and increase oxidative stress in humans, were hardly helping the American teens with acne. Since potatoes are served up mostly fried in vegetable oil, we can also consider them inflammation-promoting. American dermatologists were all wrapped up in the dietary iodine-acne connection (even though it had been debunked in 1961), while Japanese teens were enjoying small amounts of nori with their fish, as well as wakame and other seaweeds sprinkled into soups and on foods without ill effect—who knows, even with protective effects! In 1964 the Japanese were consuming about 1.20 kg of sea vegetables per person over the year—not exorbitant amounts; however, it was 1.20 kg more than Americans were eating. If seaweed and its iodine were causing acne the way some still claim it does, then obviously the rates of acne would have been much higher in the Japanese adolescents!

Knowing what we know now about milk and acne promotion, can you imagine the differences in the blood markers of acne-related hormones brought on by the massive amounts of milk consumed in the United States? Americans were consuming ten times more milk per person than the Japanese in 1964! Undoubtedly that would cause a significant difference in the blood levels of acne-promoting androgen precursors and insulin-like growth hormone. Then, of course, we have the inflammation-promoting animal (saturated) and vegetable oil fats—Americans were outnumbering their Japanese counterparts by consuming five times as much animal fat and about three times as much vegetable oil. As for insulin-spiking sweets, you really didn't think that America would play second fiddle to Japan, did you? No, once again the American consumption of sweets and sugars was more than twice that of the Japanese.

The Westernization of the Japanese diet has happened at lightning speed. New studies are showing that the blood cholesterol levels of Americans and Japanese, once a mile apart, are now only marginally different. The increase in processed food consumption in Japan has soared by well over 200 percent since 1970. The healthy intake of dietary fiber, the same fiber capable of influencing the acne-promoting hormones, has seen a 31 percent reduction since the Japanese versus American acne study of the 1960s. In a thorough review of the changing situation among Japanese children, published in the *American Journal of Clinical Nutrition* (2000), Dr. Mitsunori Murata of Tokyo Women's Medical College also noted that about 80 percent of all students in junior and senior high school have developed a sedentary lifestyle outside school. This, of course, does nothing to lower stress and inflammation, and it pushes the development of weight gain. In Japan the number of obese children increased by about 40 percent from 1976 through the year 2000. Indeed, the upward trends in the incidence of cardiovascular disease and the increases in waist circumference and body weight among urban dwellers in Japanese cities should be expected when considering the sedentary lifestyle and massive shifts in dietary quality. Men of all ages and older women have seen significant gains in body weight and a higher body mass index (BMI) over the last decade. As reported in the *Japan Times* (December 6, 2006), there are now 9.4 million Japanese with excess accumulation of abdominal fat, and an additional 10.2 million who are on the cusp. Those are actually pretty alarming numbers in a nation with a population only one-third that of the United States. The only exception is the young to middle-aged women living in Japan's largest cities who have actually seen a *decrease* in BMI over the last twenty-five years, most likely due to the tremendous social pressure for young Japanese women to remain thin.

The first American-franchised fast-food joint hung out its shingle, or we should say, arches, in 1976, and since then the fast-food industry has grown to colossal proportions—in 2003 the Japanese fast-food market was estimated at 14.8 billion (U.S.) dollars. As reported in the cover story in *New Scientist* (February 1, 2003), the combination of high fat, high sugar, and excess calories may have addictive-like properties. Whatever the case may be, it is evident that the Japanese have been lured in by this delicious, fat- and sugar-laden, potentially acne-promoting fare. These "tempting delights" are served up with a smile while the American fast-food fat cats and corporate stakeholders go laughing to the bank. Chopsticks, who needs them? The fast-food meal is starting to become the rule rather than the exception for many young Japanese, and whether truly addictive or not, they certainly keep going back for more.

Before the Western fast-food influences spread like a smallpox epidemic carried by foreigners into the region, there was the *traditional* Japanese diet. This diet is still consumed by a majority of older Japanese. Elements of the traditional Japanese diet include lots of fish and seafood, moderate soy, green tea, sesame, minimally processed foods/grains, plenty of fiber, small amounts of seaweed, and an amazing variety of colorful antioxidants from fruits and vegetables.

It is also worth making note of an item that was not a major component of the traditional Japanese diet—milk. It wasn't even a minor component of the traditional Japanese diet. Only recently have the Japanese started to indulge in large amounts of milk. Despite all the hoopla about milk and osteoporosis, it should be highlighted that the once very low rates of osteoporosis in Japan are now rapidly approaching those of North America. Evidently all those extra gallons of milk are doing little to curb an osteoporosis epidemic in Asia. As pointed out in a recent review in the journal *Pediatrics* (2005), increased consumption of dairy products has not shown even a modestly consistent benefit for child or young adult bone health. A previous investigation in the *American Journal of Clinical Nutrition* (2000) reviewed fifty-seven studies and concluded that there was inadequate evidence to support the recommendations for increased daily intake of dairy foods for bone health in the general population. The authors of the more recent *Pediatrics* study point out that there are many ways of ensuring adequate calcium intake outside dairy—dark green leafy vegetables, tofu, broccoli, sweet potatoes, instant oats, enriched cereals, soy milks, and enriched juices, to name a few sources.

The largest population studies have not shown a lower risk of fracture among those eating or drinking gallons of dairy—actually, the highest risks of fractures occur in nations with the highest consumption of dairy! The bottom line is that calcium-milk is arguably the most overstated notion in nutritional medicine. We underscore

Non-Dairy Calcium Sources

almonds	okra
bok choy	pinto beans
broccoli	red beans
Chinese cabbage	rhubarb
enriched orange juice	sardines with bones
enriched rice beverages	spinach
enriched soy milk	tofu
fortified cereals	white beans
kale	

this here because doctors with little nutritional knowledge continue to use this dairy party line. The Clear Skin Diet is a milk-restrictive diet, and with just a little effort those with acne can take steps to ensure adequate calcium intake from other sources. It is perhaps most important to consider vitamin D, an essential nutrient, and one that has been added to milk for decades. There is good evidence that the general population has an inadequate vitamin D intake, one that might be potentially compounded by milk avoidance, staying out of the sun, and using vitamin D–blocking sunscreens. While avoiding dairy, acne patients should seek out alternative beverages such as rice and soy milks that are fortified with vitamin D. Fish rich in omega-3 fatty acids are often great sources of vitamin D, as well as various mushrooms and fortified cereals. Supplementation of 400 to 800 IU may also be prudent.

Back to the Japanese diet—it is not just the nutritiously dense foods within the Japanese diet that make it so healthy, it is also the often-overlooked methods of preparation. Traditional Japanese food is consumed in the most natural way possible; for maximum flavor and nutrient value, fish is often eaten raw, and foods are minimally cooked. Until recent years most Japanese kitchens were without conventional ovens, and even though most households now have an oven, they are not used to the same degree as in Western cooking. The last time Dr. Logan spent a month with his extended Japanese family in Tokyo, the oven was not even used once for the delicious home-cooked meals. The end result is greater consumption of foods that are steamed, boiled, sautéed, or stir-fried over low heat versus long cooking times in dry-heat ovens. If you recall from chapter 3, "Dampening the Flames of Acne," the avoidance of overcooked foods prepared in high-dry heat will greatly reduce your intake of the dietary AGEs, which otherwise promote inflammation and oxidative stress throughout the body.

While the Japanese did not include much milk or dairy in the traditional diet, they historically have been massive consumers of a clear-skin beverage called green tea. More than 70 percent of older Japanese, those most likely to adhere to the traditional Japanese diet, consume green tea on a regular basis. According to a 2005 nationwide study by the American Institute of Cancer Research, the percentage of the American adult population that consumes green tea on a regular basis is only a paltry 8 percent.

While traditional Japanese meals are the opposite of supersize when it comes to portions, they are not minimized when it comes to *variety*. A recent survey showed that older Japanese women consume more than a hundred different types of food per week, while the typical Western food consumer is doing well if they hit thirty different types. In Dr. Logan's travels and experiences of traditional home cooking in Japan, he is always fascinated by how many bowls and small plates (with wide nutritional variety) can be squeezed onto the tables in Japanese homes. The traditional meal is actually made up of several small dishes at one sitting. It is not uncommon to have six or seven different small plates and bowls in front of you while dining, each one comprising many different food components. Since dietary anti-oxidants work together in a synergistic fashion, the varied traditional Japanese diet allows greater opportunity for protective synergy.

Since the rates of acne in Japan are now indistinguishable from those in the United States and other nations consuming the processed Westernized diet, it is clear that something happened along the way between 1964 and today. It could be argued that the modern lifestyle in Japan is a more sedentary and stressful one, and this could certainly be a player in promoting acne. However, knowing what we know now about nutritional influences on hormonal-related illness, inflammation, and oxidative stress, it would be naïve to suggest that the massive dietary changes in Japan have nothing to do with the rise in acne.

It is also noteworthy that there were increases in the rates of male-pattern baldness (androgenetic alopecia) among Japanese men in the latter half of the twentieth century. Dr. Masumi Inaba, a leading physician and surgeon in Japan, was convinced that the phenomenon of increasing baldness was due in part to the large-scale dietary changes, particularly in genetically susceptible individuals. This proposed diet-baldness connection is mentioned here because there is a well-documented overlap between the hormones that stoke the fires of acne and those that promote baldness in adult males (and females). For example, the conversion of testosterone into the potent acne hormone dihydrotestosterone by $5\alpha R$ is also at work in thinning out the hairs on top of the head. Dr. Inabi had some of his work translated into English, including his work *Can Human Hair Grow Again?* (Azabu

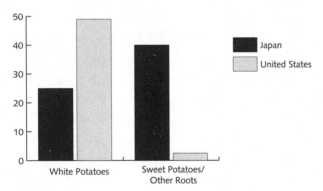

Annual consumption of white potatoes vs. sweet potatoes, yams, and other roots in kilograms per person, 1964.

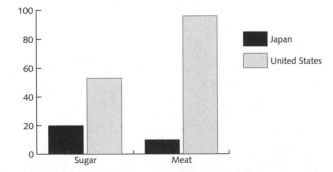

Annual consumption of sugar and meat in kilograms per person, 1964.

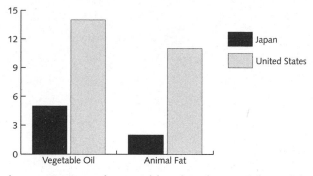

Annual consumption of vegetable oil and animal fat in kilograms per person, 1964.

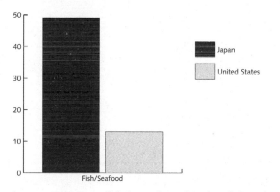

Annual consumption of fish and seafood in kilograms per person, 1964.

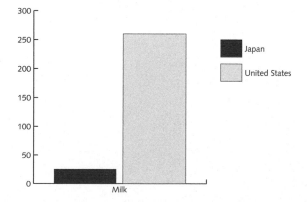

Annual consumption of milk in kilograms per person, 1964.

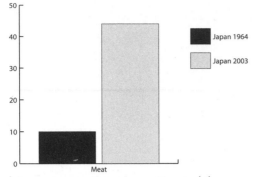

Annual Japanese meat consumption in kilograms per person—then vs. now.

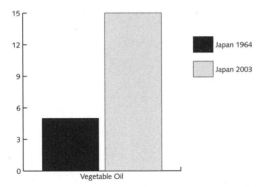

Annual Japanese vegetable oil consumption in kilograms per person—then vs. now.

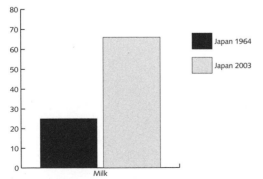

Annual Japanese milk consumption in kilograms per person—then vs. now.

Shokan Publishing, 1985). Here he points a causal finger at the Western diet, with too much meat/animal fats, too much sugar and high-fat dairy products, a lack of fish and healthy seaweeds, too many acidic foods/not enough alkaline fruits and vegetables, and not enough whole grains. Dr. Inaba was a mainstream doctor, not some alternative medicine maverick; he was awarded the highest medal of merit for his work by the Japan Medical Association in 1979. He was also way ahead of his time in the arena of nutritional medicine.

The Japanese experience, and what can only be described as one of the largest nutritional experiments ever conducted, speaks loudly to the acne-diet connection. We highlight it in *The Clear Skin Diet* because it represents in simple terms the lessons of clear skin through nutrition. We are not suggesting that the nutritional path to clear skin is only through the mandatory use of chopsticks and the consumption of raw fish. We would like you to examine the graphs that follow and look for the dietary excesses that have occurred at the expense of high-quality nutritional foods. At the same time, also consider the importance of minimally processed foods and the value of variety; this is the true essence of the traditional, acne-protective Japanese diet.

8

Action Plan for the Clear Skin Diet

OKAY, SO THE BOOK IS called *The Clear Skin Diet*, which might imply that we are only concerned with diet and healthy skin. However, with all of our diversions into stress, exercise, and relaxation, you may have already figured out that there is a little more to clear skin than diet alone—truthfully, the book could have been called *The Clear Skin Lifestyle*. In the following pages we will discuss the Action Plan for the Clear Skin Diet, the real operating plan for clear skin. This is what it boils down to: taking action to support your overall health and improving your chances of healthy, glowing skin, while reducing and eliminating acne lesions. The background is done, we have taken you through the twists and turns of the history surrounding the diet-stress-lifestyle and acne connections, we have also discussed the eye-opening research that signals the dawning of a new era in holistic or integrative dermatology. All of this might be great information; however, like any other nutrition and lifestyle book, without application it will just sit on a dusty shelf and remain just that—stored information. Now is the time to roll up your sleeves and make the changes that will ultimately become part of your habits, and your lifestyle.

Your Action Plan includes four parts:

      1. *Sleep*

      2. *Relaxation Response*

      3. *Exercise*

      4. *Diet*

Yes, diet is, of course, in the Action Plan, and we will certainly provide the key dietary principles to lower sebum production, prevent rises in acne-related hormones, limit inflammation, and protect against free-radical damage. However, we will emphasize the other lifestyle factors first, because our experience shows that when these are perfected, the dietary changes that support clear skin are greatly accelerated. While some will want to plunge immediately into all aspects of the Action Plan, this is not a necessity. Most will find it more practical, and perhaps more rewarding, to take it one or two steps at a time. Each time you embark on a new step, commit to it for three months, or ninety days if you prefer it that way. We have never been impressed by these weekly or monthly books and plans that make all sorts of promises for acne and other aspects of health. Studies within behavioral medicine show that if you keep up with a lifestyle change for three months, you have a better chance of making it a habit. While the anti-inflammatory benefits induced by dietary changes may be noticed in visible acne within a shorter period of time, it is also important to reconsider our previous discussions on comedo formation—this process can take months! Therefore, the preventative nature of the diet may take months to truly notice. Time and commitment to the Clear Skin Lifestyle are essential for significant progress.

It is important to provide yourself with an assessment of your starting point, your baseline. Dr. Treloar has prepared the Clear Skin Diet Assessment Form, which gives you (and your health-care provider) a synopsis of where you are at the starting blocks. Before delving into the Action Plan, this worksheet will provide a rapid assessment of how significant your acne is, the state of affairs of your typical diet, your stressors, the psychological impact of acne, your physical activity, sleep, and, for women, the menstrual markers that may be significant to the picture. The Clear Skin Diet Assessment

Form is available for download in a printer-friendly format at Dr. Treloar's website: www.integrativederm.com. The form is not only a baseline assessment; filled out on a regular basis, it also provides a means to assess progress along the way toward clear skin. By using the Clear Skin Diet Worksheet, you can easily determine how your acne condition, stress, dietary habits, sleep, and exercise are changing as you make progress. The companion form that follows, the Clear Skin Diet Diary, will help you adhere to the Action Plan for success.

Record keeping is a key to the success of the Action Plan, so keep a journal or, at the very least, remember to complete your daily copy of Dr. Treloar's preprepared copy of the Clear Skin Diet Diary, which follows. This form is available for downloading in a printer-friendly format at Dr. Treloar's website: www.integrativederm.com. Maintaining such a diary has been proven to increase your chances of success when it comes to behavioral changes.

The Clear Skin Diet Diary is central to the Action Plan because it serves as a reality check. Taking the time to fill it out will force you to question yourself on your daily sleep, exercise, relaxation, and, yes, as its name implies, diet is also queried. Research consistently shows that we humans tend to believe we eat healthier than we really do, and that we are more physically active than we really are. For example, a large national Canadian survey found that three-quarters of the population believed they ate a nutritious and balanced diet, yet in the same survey only one out of six met even the minimum recommendations for consumption of fruits and vegetables (*Globe & Mail*, July 5, 2002, Andre Picard). Keeping the Clear Skin Diet Diary will provide a clear view of reality and will promote your adherence to the Action Plan as you move toward clear skin. So make ninety copies, bind them, and keep them in a readily accessible place.

Action Plan Part One: Sleep

We have mentioned sleep a number of times throughout the book, particularly in the context of stress. While there isn't much research in the area of sleep and its direct influence on the progression of acne, international studies do show that patients frequently report that lack of proper sleep aggravates acne. This is not entirely surprising since

The Clear Skin Diet Assessment

Name _____ birthdate _____ m/f _____ date _____

Age at which acne appeared/worsened _____

Distribution of acne   back chest forehead cheeks nose chin neck

Type of acne lesions   comedones papules pustules nodules scars

Degree of acne   mild   moderate   severe

Sleep   hours per night _____   interruptions per night _____

          for what reasons? _____

Psychological impact of acne   none 1 2 3 4 5 6 7 8 9 10 unbearable

Stress   none 1 2 3 4 5 6 7 8 9 10 unbearable

   Reasons _____

Exercise   Strength training ____   times per week _____ duration _____

             Flexibility ____   times per week _____ duration _____

             Cardiovascular ____   times per week _____ duration _____

Stress Management/
Relaxation Response Activity _____   times per week _____ duration _____

Bowel movements per week _____

Typical diet   vegetables   fruit   carbohydrates   protein   fat   sweets

   breakfast _____

   snack   _____

   lunch   _____

   snack   _____

   dinner   _____

   snack   _____

Cups per day

   milk _____   beer/wine/liquor _____

   soda _____   fruit juice _____

   coffee/tea _____   vegetable juice _____

- -

Women only

   Unwanted facial hair _____

   Birth control pills _____

   Menstrual cycle: regular   irregular   bloating

                breast tenderness   perimenstrual acne flare   mood changes

The Clear Skin Diet Diary

Day # _____

Day & date _____

Cycle Day* _____ (first day of bleeding counts as day 1)

Sleep   hours last night _____   interruptions last night _____

for what reasons?_____

Stress levels   none 1 2 3 4 5 6 7 8 9 10 unbearable

Relaxation response activity   _____ duration _____

Exercise   Strength training _____   duration _____

Flexibility _____   duration _____

Cardiovascular _____   duration _____

Diet   vegetables   fruit   carbohydrates   protein   fat   wish I hadn't

breakfast _____

snack _____

lunch _____

snack _____

dinner _____

snack _____

milk _____   beer/wine/liquor _____

soda _____   fruit juice _____

coffee/tea _____   vegetable juice _____

Moved bowels _____

Acne (new lesions today)

	papules	pustules	comedones	nodules
face	_____	_____	_____	_____
chest	_____	_____	_____	_____
back	_____	_____	_____	_____
_____	_____	_____	_____	_____

*Women only

inadequate sleep disturbs your adrenal gland function and increases levels of cortisol. Remember cortisol? It is the stress hormone that has been shown to be elevated in acne patients and the very same hormone that increases your tendency to become insulin resistant. The emerging research shows that the nasty side effects of too much insulin hanging around include the promotion of acne. Sleep deprivation also changes how we eat—it promotes the intake of excess calories, more fats, and sugars, and less healthy fruits and vegetables. To top it off, sleep deprivation just feels awful. So we have the reasons for promoting sleep to promote clear skin, and now here is the plan.

ACTION PLAN FOR GOOD SLEEP HABITS

* Devote the time to sleep. Arrange consistent bedtimes and waking times to allow seven to eight hours of uninterrupted sleep.
* Begin unwinding thirty to forty-five minutes before sleep should begin. Do not use this time to stimulate your mind with to-do lists, task completions, house cleaning, etc.
* If you have worries, write them down and leave them for tomorrow.
* Practice the Relaxation Response, meditation, and other mind-body medicine techniques before bed.
* Avoid daytime naps.
* Bedroom should be quiet.
* Bedroom should be as dark as possible for maximum melatonin release.
* Bedroom should be used for sleeping and sex only. Remove the television and computer—viewed late at night, they may negatively influence melatonin levels.
* Bedroom environment should be organized and free of clutter; it should be an oasis from the rest of the world.
* Bedroom temperature should be comfortable—too much heat interferes with sleep.
* Keep a regular schedule; go to bed as close to the same time every night as possible.
* Eliminate/reduce caffeine-containing beverages in the evening.
* Perform your regular, moderate physical activity/exercise in the daytime or early evening.

✖ Alcohol should not be used as a sleep aid; avoid it four to six hours before bed.

✖ Avoid eating large meals and lots of fluids before bed.

✖ Try drinking a small amount of rice beverage and/or eating a small piece of whole grain toast before bedtime.

✖ Consider a few drops of quality lavender or jasmine on a hand-kerchief under the pillow.

✖ Keep your cellphone away from the bedside—it may have a negative influence on melatonin and sleep quality.

✖ Consider a bedtime ritual, such as a warm bath or a few pages of reading.

Action Plan Part Two: Relaxation Response

Most diet and nutritional medicine books tend to view food consumption in isolation, without consideration for the psychosocial context in which food is consumed. As we discussed in chapter 6, "The Brain-Skin Connection," psychological stress can have a profound influence on acne itself, as well as our dietary choices. Therefore, the Action Plan for the Clear Skin Diet emphasizes the induction of the relaxation response and techniques used to manage stress. The healing and stress-reducing relaxation response can be induced by many of the techniques of mind-body medicine we described and outlined in chapter 6—meditation, hypnotherapy, biofeedback, guided imagery and visualization, yoga, prayer, tai chi, breathing exercises, therapeutic writing, art, music, and dance. The cognitive-behavioral interventions we described can be very valuable in stress reduction.

You can choose from the buffet of choices to lower stress. However, it is important to point out that you don't need to pay big bucks to "the best" yoga instructor to turn on your innate relaxation response. It really doesn't take much of your time, and the financial cost to turn on the relaxation response and turn down the dial on stress can be free. What it does require is consistent practice to become proficient. The payoff is huge because you have a portable stress reducer that is ready in virtually all situations. Extensive work by Dr. Herbert Benson and colleagues from Harvard has revealed that the relaxation response can be induced by the following;

1. A quiet, comfortable environment, with you in a comfortable position

2. Conscious relaxation of the muscles of the body

3. Repetition of a simple mental stimulus such as a word, phrase, image, or prayer

4. A passive mental attitude toward the process itself and any intrusive sounds or thoughts

5. Duration of ten to twenty minutes

What we know about the relaxation response is that both the mind and the body are calmed, which in turn can recondition a more appropriate response to stressors. The relaxation response reduces arousal in the emotional center of the brain called the limbic system. This, in turn, leads to a reduction of stress-related hormones such as epinephrine and the acne-related hormone cortisol. Of course, lower stress and lower cortisol may lead to a decreased storage of abdominal fat and more appropriate food choices.

The regular practice of the relaxation response can reduce overactivity of the stress branch of the nervous system, and, over time, it can lower the threat level perceived by stress-prone individuals. Research published by Dr. Benson of Harvard, and colleagues from other universities around the world, has shown that the relaxation response is helpful in many stress-related conditions. The effects of the relaxation response have now been confirmed using sophisticated brain-imaging studies.

Consider also your social support and your affiliation with others; this is very important in resilience to life's stressors. Quite often we get what we give, so continue to work at being a good friend and express your love daily to strengthen the social bonds. Other techniques to reduce stress that we emphasize as part of the Action Plan include assertiveness (learning to say "no"), time management, organization, realistic expectations, needs assessments, letting go of perfectionism, and using humor to your advantage. These are reviewed in the Action Plan—Relaxation Response, which follows.

Remember that stress-management techniques and the value of the relaxation response are not substitutes for appropriate mental-health evaluation and care. If you have psychological issues or problems related to your acne or otherwise, please seek professional evaluation, counseling, and therapy.

ACTION PLAN—RELAXATION RESPONSE

✖ Choose from the buffet of mind-body medicine and daily practice of Dr. Benson's relaxation response.

✖ Awareness of life events—mindfulness—keep track of stressors when completing Dr. Treloar's Clear Skin Diet Diary. Make efforts to limit the buildup of stress. Ask yourself, "Do I really need this?"—referring, of course, to the source of stress.

✖ Organize and Prioritize—minimize clutter in your home, work, and mind.

✖ Manage Your Time—choose tasks and activities with care; prioritize and complete tasks in order of importance and one at a time.

✖ Let Go of Perfectionism—Don't sweat the small stuff.

✖ Be Assertive—Learn to say no and ask for help to prevent overload.

✖ Humor—Laugh and love every day.

Action Plan Part Three: Exercise

If exercise were a pill, doctors would prescribe it to everyone. Proper, moderate exercise performed in a safe manner helps to control insulin, reduce stress, lift depression, alleviate anxiety, and improve sleep and overall body composition. On the other hand, according to research published in *Cancer Epidemiology Biomarkers and Prevention* (2003), being a couch potato is associated with increased levels of IGF-1, the acne-promoting hormone. Exercise, therefore, has the potential to help acne patients through a number of mechanisms.

Our physiologic response to stress, the rapid increase in the sympathetic nervous system, is called the fight-or-flight response. It prepares our body to respond to a perceived threat by ramping up the blood flow to our muscles, increasing our heart rate and blood pressure—in other words, we are ready and set to go for what could be considered vigorous exercise. Too bad we can't pop into the gym immediately after the boss upsets us in an unpleasant meeting or when that wacky driver cuts us off in traffic. Well, you don't always need a formal gym setting. You could consider doing what experts call "exercise snacks"—these can be anything from pacing while talking on the phone, choosing the farthest parking spot rather than "stressing" over finding a close spot, choosing stairs over elevators and escalators, exiting one subway station away from work, or intentionally spending time walking during a coffee break at work. The list of potential exercise snacks is virtually endless. In a world set up for convenience, we must be mindful of physical activity and intentionally go out of our way to exercise.

You might be tempted to say that you really don't have time to exercise, and both of us have heard that excuse many times. The reality is that everyone has the time to exercise; it's a matter of making time and using time management wisely. Consider that research shows *no difference* in leisure-time physical activity between those who work thirty-five or fewer hours and those who work fifty-plus hours per week.

In addition to the exercise snacks, you can participate in formal exercise plans which should be part of your routine. Exercise comes in three forms: aerobic exercise, strength training, and flexibility/stretching exercises. Aerobic exercise is generally of longer duration and uses oxygen in the energy-generating process at the muscular level. Examples include walking, swimming, jogging, playing tennis, and soccer. Strength training is anaerobic (without the use of oxygen in the energy-generating process) and involves shorter bursts of intense exercise to maintain lean muscle mass. Examples include lifting dumbbells or performing other weight-bearing exercises and resistance training. Stretching/flexibility exercises improve range of motion, mobility, and the ability to perform both aerobic and anaerobic activities. Examples include an overhead reach with both arms, rotating and stretching while seated in a chair, and raising the legs while lying down. All three are important, and the strength training and aerobic exercises should be alternated most days of the week for around thirty to forty minutes per session. The flexibility exercises can be incorporated into your relaxation response plan or in conjunction with your regular exercise routine.

Ensure that you obtain the all-clear from your doctor before you begin an exercise routine. If you can afford one, a professional trainer can be helpful, especially in the early going through that ninety-day period we talked about for habit forming. This is the time when guidance, support, and structure can facilitate proper technique and adherence to the plan.

We should also warn against overtraining and exhaustive exercise. Research shows that not only can excess strenuous exercise cause physical harm, it can also lead to an elevated stress response, stress hormones, and subsequent psychological problems. The key is in moderate exercise that makes you feel good. After the first few weeks, if you are reacting with exhaustion, a lowered mood, and waking up feeling unrefreshed, chances are you are doing too much.

ACTION PLAN—EXERCISE

* ✖ Do something, an intentional session of physical activity, for ten to forty minutes once or twice daily
* ✖ Walk whenever you can.
* ✖ Consider your "exercise snacks." Be mindful of opportunities to trade convenience for physical activity.
* ✖ Include aerobic and strength training for twenty minutes or so at least two to three times weekly, and flexibility or calming exercises for ten to thirty minutes daily for a complete, balanced plan.
* ✖ Keep your diary to check yourself and your adherence to the plan.
* ✖ "No time" is not an acceptable excuse.
* ✖ Work with a professional if possible to get started.

Action Plan Part Four: Diet

Ah, yes, the diet plan! We could leave it at the advice of science journalist Michael Pollan, who provided the most abbreviated version of the healthy diet in the *New York Times Magazine* (Unhappy Meals, January 28, 2007): "Eat food. Not much. Mostly plants." We love this line; however, the Action Plan for the Clear Skin Diet is just a little more complex, and yet with minimal effort it can easily become a habit-forming way to help reduce and prevent acne.

The Action Plan is a diet of both inclusion and exclusion/limitation—some foods promote the acne process through inflammation, oxidative stress, hormonal imbalance and blood-sugar spiking. On the other hand, the intake of certain foods should be prioritized, for they are able to suppress inflammation, support the antioxidant defense system, regulate hormones, and balance blood sugar. You probably found that we extolled the same nutrients again and again in chapter after chapter, their benefits derived from a few different mechanisms. Certain foods kept on making our "bad food" list, once again through various mechanisms. We acknowledge that we did not approach this book in a superficial way, and the reading at times may have been scientifically deep; however, understanding the acne causes and pathways allows us to understand how nutrition can put a dent in the process. All of the twists and turns in *The Clear Skin Diet* have converged to intersect into the pathological mechanisms of acne.

ACTION PLAN PART FOUR—DIET

✖ Keep your blood sugar and insulin levels balanced by eating nutrient-dense meals and mini-meals every two and a half to three hours. This will help control cravings, making it easier for you to nurture yourself with good stuff and avoid impulse eating. Avoid unhealthy processed, sugary, and fatty snacks. Think about fruit and whole grain.

✖ Make every effort to be mindful about your eating experience, and try to eat in what you perceive to be a relaxed and pleasurable setting. Start your meal with a momentary pause of appreciation. Enjoy your foods and appreciate your dining companions.

Foods to Include:

✖ Produce—and lots of it.

Vegetables, vegetables, and more vegetables—including sea vegetables. Consume a minimum of five servings of deeply colored fruits and vegetables daily. Follow the rainbow and choose a variety of reds, oranges, yellows, greens, blues, and purples.

Fruit, especially berries and grapefruit. Use caution with fruits that carry a high concentration of sugar such as banana, watermelon, and raisins.

✖ Protein

Fish, especially oily wild caught and small fish such as sardines, anchovies, and mackerel. Canned wild salmon is an easy option. High quality fish oil capsules should be considered (see the appendix).

Lean meat and poultry, especially grass-fed or free range. Consider limiting red meat to once per week.

Eggs, particularly high omega-3 from free range, cage-free chickens.

Soy—in moderation, especially fermented soy such as miso and tempeh.

✖ Carbohydrates

Whole grains—take a little extra time to cook brown rice, quinoa, buckwheat, bulgar, barley.

Breads and pastas should be limited and enjoyed in the whole grain form.

Don't forget vegetable carbohydrates including squash, sweet potato, and green beans.

✖ Fats/Oils

Extra virgin olive oil, canola oil, rice bran oil, omega-3-rich oils (flaxseed and walnut as dressings) not for cooking, small amounts of sesame oil for flavor and antioxidants.

✖ Spices and Herbs

Ginger, turmeric, and cinnamon.

✖ Lacto-fermented Foods

Unsweetened yogurt*, kefir*, sauerkraut, kimchee, unpasteurized pickled vegetables

✖ Nuts*

✖ These are subject to the personal sensitivities of biochemical individuality. Experiment with them and beware allergy, exacerbation of, acne, and indigestibility. Brining and toasting as described in the recipe section may help with digestive tolerability. Brazil nuts are very high in selenium; two or three per day is more than enough.

✖ Beverages

Green tea, tomato, and 100 percent vegetable juices (watch the sodium!); consider investing in your own juice maker for home. Kombucha fermented "tea" with a refreshing vinegary flavor.

✖ Daily Multivitamin-Mineral Formula

See the appendix for high quality recommendations.

FOODS TO LIMIT*

✖ Produce

Fruits—use caution with those that are dense in sugar such as bananas, watermelon, and dried fruits. Berries have a very low Glycemic Index (GI) and are less likely to spike blood sugar.

Vegetables—Use caution with starchy vegetables, particularly with the skin removed (e.g. mashed white potatoes) the higher GI can spike blood sugar.

✖ Protein

Fish containing high mercury and environmental toxins. (See our discussion on pages 66–67 and www.ewg.org.)

High AGE foods, particularly meats with sugar, glaze or marinades cooked on high heat in the absence of moisture.

Full fat cheeses.**

Processed meats and cheese.

✖ Carbohydrates

"High-Glycemic" choices that are concentrated in sugar and low in fiber.

White rice, mashed potatoes, white breads, and pasta; baked goods that are processed, high in sugar, and cooked on high, dry heat (high GI and high AGE).

High-sugar, dairy-based products that are unfermented, e.g., sherbet, ice cream, milk chocolate.**

✖ Fats/Oils

Omega-6-rich oils—corn, safflower, sunflower, soybean oils. Look for them in prepared meals, baked goods and in animal products where these oils were fed during growth.

Saturated fats—butter and lard.

✖ Beverages

Soft drinks, soda, undiluted fruit juices

Alcoholic beverages

Milk**

FOODS TO EXCLUDE—PSEUDOFOODS

✖ Man-made fats and oils—hydrogenated vegetable oils/trans fats

✖ Margarine

✖ Vegetable oils heated to very high temperatures for fried foods and oils that have been used multiple times for cooking

✖ Artificial sweeteners, food colors and preservatives

✖ High-fructose corn syrup

Tips: Work with a nutritionally oriented doctor or nutritionist to get started. They can help you find ways to bring these foods into (and out of) your life. A good nutritionist will also be an excellent freelance coach and cheerleader.

See Dr. Gabriella Chow's excellent recipes and the tips from nutritionist Kristine Bahr provided in chapter 9, and remember that we tend to eat what is around us—if you stock ice cream, pastries, and fatty chips as snack foods, chances are that is what you will eat at grazing time. On the other hand, if what is available includes healthy snacks of whole fruit and whole grains low in fat and sugar and higher in fiber, you will reach for these items.

*Biochemical Individuality—dermatologists have acknowledged for years that individual patients may negatively react to certain foods or dietary components. Individual genetic variations in metabolic processing may be at work. Some patients may see an aggravation from nuts, while others may not. The same is true of dairy, sugar dense fruits, soybean oil, or any other foods we listed in the Foods to Limit section. We encourage personal experimentation; you might find that certain foods and/or dietary components are absolute acne aggravators and that they must be placed in the Foods to Exclude category.

**Dairy-Free for Life? Maintaining a dairy-free diet can be difficult for many patients because milk, cream, and other dairy foods find their way into so many foods. Based on the recommendations of Dr. William Danby, an expert in this area, we encourage a three month trial of a dairy-free diet. After this time you can evaluate your progress and experiment with various dairy-based yogurts with live active bacterial cultures.

The Clear Skin Diet on One Page

Open & Closed Comedones Papules & Pustules	Normal Pilosebaceous Unit Clear Skin
Genetics	Genetics
High stress/poor sleep	Stress management/sleep
Sedentary lifestyle	Regular exercise
Insulin-spiking sweets/carbohydrates	Fiber-rich foods
High omega-6 fats	High omega-3 fats
High saturated/trans fats	Low saturated/trans fats
Lack deeply colored veggies	Deeply colored veggies
Milk	No milk
Soft drinks	Green tea
No lycopene	Tomatoes/tomato juice
No culinary variety	Ginger-turmeric
Excess animal meats	Fish, fermented soy
Unbalanced intestinal bacteria	Healthy intestinal bacteria

The Clear Skin Diet Recipes

BEFORE PRESENTING A VARIETY OF recipes, we have some practical tips from noted expert nutritionist Kristine Bahr. We are thrilled to have Kristine's contribution and guidance on menu planning and snacks, two very important considerations in maintaining the Clear Skin Diet. For more on Kristine and her expertise, please visit www.nutritional-balance.com.

Tips from the Nutritionist

There's a reason the party always ends up in the kitchen. Sure, it's where we find the food, but it's also the most comfortable place in the house. Both our bodies and our souls find nourishment in the kitchen. If you set aside an hour to devote to meal preparation and spend a few minutes a week planning, you will find cooking itself to be nurturing, too, rather than rushed and stressful. If your schedule does not give you an hour before dinnertime, you may find it easier to do your prep in the evening or early in the morning. Some of us revere the slow cooker; others cook in quantity and freeze so we have fast, good meals. We all spend lots of time cleaning and cutting vegetables! But it all comes down to this: to eat well, we must cook.

Tools for the kitchen include:
- chef's knife with a non-serrated blade, 6–8 inches long
- paring knife
- cutting board
- blender and/or food processor
- colander/strainer
- salad spinner
- vegetable brush for cleaning fruits and vegetables
- steamer basket to go inside a saucepan
- measuring cups and spoons
- medium frying pan or sauté pan
- large- and medium-sized saucepans
- large and small mixing bowls
- glass storage containers with lids in several different sizes
- spatula
- scraper
- kitchen scissors
- tongs
- large spoons

The following are nice to have:
- pressure cooker
- dehydrator
- steamer
- mandoline slicer
- mixer
- slow cooker
- stockpot

Also, always buy good quality glass, ceramic, and/or stainless steel products. Avoid plastic and aluminum.

We highly recommend filtering your drinking and cooking water. If you can afford it, consider filtering your bath water, too. Explore bottled waters as a treat. Look for glass bottles and try special mineral waters such as Gerolsteiner or San Pellegrino.

Clean out your cupboards and refrigerator: read the labels and discard foods that contain hydrogenated oils, artificial sweeteners, and fructose, especially high-fructose corn syrup. You may be surprised at how quickly your trash barrel fills and how empty your cupboards look after this exercise. See our shopping list for how to restock, but go slowly. Introduce new foods a few at a time. Do not overwhelm yourself.

WASH FRUITS AND VEGETABLES

Soak fruits and vegetables for ten minutes in a sinkful of water containing one of the following: ½ cup white vinegar, 4 teaspoons of salt and the juice from two or three lemons, or 10 drops grapefruit seed extract per ounce of water.

SNACKS ARE GOOD FOR YOU

Yes, we want you to eat them. Eating every two to three hours helps keep the blood sugar and insulin levels even. However, healthy snacks can be a challenge, so we have compiled a list of some of the best.

- Crudités (good old raw, chopped veggies to eat with your fingers). Clean and cut into sticks, slices, chunks, rounds, slivers, or ribbons . . . or don't bother cutting. Spend fifteen minutes filling a few jars with a variety of veggies. Put a few ice cubes on top and stow in the fridge for quick snacking. Array on a platter, salt lightly, and watch them disappear. Favorites include carrots, celery, peppers (green, red, yellow, orange), cucumber, tomatoes (cherry, grape), radishes, daikon, scallions, kohlrabi, sunchokes, turnip, jicama, zucchini, and lightly steamed green beans, peapods, broccoli, cauliflower, and asparagus.

- Dips for crudités include bean dips, yogurt/mayo dips, potato dips, spinach dip, artichoke dip, pestos, tapenades, hummus, egg salad, tuna salad, chicken salad, sardine spread, BLT dip (recipes follow).

- Marinated veggies: Mix in a jar with a screw-top lid: ½ cup olive oil, 1 tablespoon capers, 1 or 2 whole peeled garlic cloves, ¼ cup white wine or rice vinegar, and a few red pepper flakes. Bring 2 quarts of lightly salted water to a boil and cook veggies in batches until tender-crisp—for example: 1 cup peeled carrots cut into rounds or little cylinders, 2 cups cauliflower cut into little "trees," 1 cup celery cut into 1–2 inch chunks. Shake the jar to mix the dressing. Place veggies in a large bowl and add ½ cup mixed types of imported pitted olives and the dressing. Toss to coat.

- Crispy beans and/or peas: Drain and rinse canned chickpeas, canellini beans, black-eyed peas, and/or black beans. Pat dry with a towel. Mix with 1–2 teaspoons olive oil. Toss with 1 teaspoon mixed spices/salt per two cans of beans (try paprika and salt OR chili powder and garlic salt OR cumin and turmeric and salt OR cracked black pepper and salt). Spread in a thin layer on a rimmed baking sheet and toast in 300° oven for about 30 minutes, shaking every 10–15 minutes until lightly browned and crispy. Store in a tightly covered container. Serving size: ¼ cup.

- Crispy nuts and/or seeds: Place raw walnuts, pecans, almonds, hazelnuts, macadamia nuts, pepitas, and/or sunflower seeds in a bowl and cover with brine. (Dissolve one rounded teaspoon of salt per cup of cold water to make brine.) Soak for 8–12 hours (longer for larger nuts). Drain. Spread nuts/seeds in a single layer on rimmed baking sheets and dry in 150° oven for 12–24 hours until crispy (longer for larger nuts). Just before you put them in the oven, you can sprinkle spices over the nuts/seeds as you did for the crispy beans/peas. Store in tightly covered containers. Serving size: ¼ cup.

- Celery stalks stuffed with nut butter or goat cheese: Consider adding chives, poppy seeds, sesame seeds, oregano, pepper, etc. to goat cheese/nut butter.

- Cooked edamame in the pod: Don't eat the pods.

- Baked chips (corn, brown rice, or potato) with bean dip/hummus, salsa, and/or guacamole or any of the dips noted above.

- Apple or pear with one tablespoon nut butter or goat cheese: Try coring the fruit, sprinkling the cut surface with lemon juice, and stuffing with the nut butter/cheese. Put a few sunflower seeds over the sticky ends. Or slice the fruit and make teeny sandwiches.

- Half a baked white or sweet potato, some of the center removed, mixed with 1–2 tablespoons of feta or goat cheese and replaced.

- Sheep's milk yogurt (Old Chatham): Mix ¾ cup with ¼ cup crispy nuts or 2–3 apricots or ¼ cup applesauce or ½ to 1 cup berries and manchego or goat cheese or feta.

- One small whole-wheat tortilla with ¼ cup feta or goat cheese or manchego crumbled over 2 tablespoons slivered onions and/or green pepper or diced tomato or avocado, toasted/broiled/grilled to soften onions and melt cheese. You can fold this in half to make a quesadilla. Good leftovers for snacking later.

- One hard boiled egg and Finn crisp crackers. Can make egg salad with a teaspoon of canola mayo and sprinklings of salt, pepper, chives, parsley, paprika, finely diced celery, or onion.

- Cucumber slices can carry all kinds of toppers. Cut on a diagonal to get a larger oval of cuke. Top with feta, goat cheese, manchego, nut butter, thin slices of leftover chicken, pork, beef, egg salad, or sardines.

- Drain and mix sardines in water or olive oil with 1–2 teaspoons canola mayo or butter to make a smooth spread. Try adding lemon zest and pepper. Spread on cucumber slices or Finn crisp or other whole-grain crackers or stuff into celery stalks.

- Grapefruit half. Have some nuts or sheep cheese or sheep yogurt to add protein to this snack.

- One-half avocado filled with 2 tablespoons canned shrimp, crabmeat, or tuna.

- One orange and ¼ cup crispy nuts.

- Corn tortilla toasted in a skillet until pliable rolled around diced tomato and feta or sliced onion and goat cheese or olives and manchego or hummus and lettuce, etc.

- Popcorn: ½–1 cup mixed with ¼ cup crispy nuts or 1–2 tablespoons diced feta or manchego cheese.

- Fresh rolls: These are a lot of work, but so yummy. Set up the ingredients. Prepare bowls containing: shredded cabbage or lettuce, radishes and/or cucumber cut in matchsticks, mint leaves, sesame seeds or chopped crispy nuts, cooked chicken breast cut in 2-inch by ½-inch pieces and/or cooked shrimp, softened cellophane rice noodles. One at a time soften 8-inch diameter "spring roll skins" in a bowl of hot water. (Spring roll skins look like thin, translucent plastic discs. They have other names including rice paper, gallette de riz and banh trang.) Spread the wiggly sheet on a clean counter and in the center place a pinch each of lettuce/cabbage, radish/cuke, seeds/nuts, rice noodles. Put a few mint leaves and a piece of chicken and/or shrimp on top. Fold the sheet up from the bottom and over the filling. Fold the sides in toward the center over the filling. Roll up, finishing with the free end of the sheet wrapped around to seal the roll. Store in the fridge wrapped in plastic wrap or covered with a damp towel. Dip in a sauce made of 1–2 tablespoons each of soy sauce and vinegar and a spot of molasses or honey. You can make these using lightly steamed cabbage leaves instead of the rice papers.

- Dips

  Bean dips, hummus, tapenade, pesto—buy these! Check the ingredients; look for canola or olive oil, avoid sugars and preservatives.

  White bean dip: Drain a can of white beans, rinse, and put through a blender or food processor with one garlic clove, black pepper, 1–2 teaspoons of olive oil, and lemon juice or vinegar. You can add oregano or thyme or tarragon.

  Potato dips: Use cooked, mashed white or sweet potatoes in place of beans.

  Hummus: Drain a can of chickpeas, rinse, and put through a blender or food processor with one garlic clove (if you roast the garlic first it mellows the flavor), 2 tablespoons of sesame tahini, 2 teaspoons of olive oil, 2 teaspoons of lemon juice, lemon zest, black pepper.

  Tapenade: Remove seeds from calamata olives and blend to a paste. May add garlic.

  Pesto: Combine in a food processor 4 cups basil leaves, 1–2 peeled garlic cloves, ¼ cup grated parmesan, ¼ cup pine nuts, 3–4 tablespoons olive oil.

Yogurt/mayo dips: In a blender mix equal parts yogurt and canola mayo with herbs of your choice such as garlic, scallion, lemon zest. (You can make a thicker dip if you make "yogurt cheese." Put yogurt in a filter in a strainer and let the whey drip through. After a few hours, the thick yogurt cheese remains in the filter.)

Spinach dip: Add chopped spinach to the yogurt/mayo dip. Add nutmeg. You can use frozen spinach, but thaw it first and press it in a towel to remove excess liquid.

Artichoke dip: Start with yogurt/mayo basic and blend in a jar of marinated artichoke hearts.

Egg, tuna, chicken, sardine salad dips just need to be finely diced in order to be dippable.

BLT dip: Combine shredded lettuce, finely diced tomatoes, and minced cooked bacon with enough canola mayo to bind.

SHOPPING LIST

VEGETABLES

Buy enough to have vegetables with every meal and snack.
Eat colorful foods from the whole spectrum of the rainbow!
Try something new every week—use the Internet to find recipes.
Don't forget sprouts.
Alliums every week (onions, leeks, scallions, shallots, garlic)
Eat crucifers every week (broccoli, cauliflower, Brussels sprouts, cabbages, radishes, kale, collards, kohlrabi).
Avocados also qualify as healthy fats.

FRUIT

Aim for 2–3 servings of fruit daily.
Explore new fruits.
lemons for juice and peel

PROTEIN

fish once or twice a week
lean beef
lean pork

Sample Menus

Day	Breakfast	Lunch	Dinner
1	Eggs (2) scrambled with peppers/onions/tomatoes using 2 teaspoons of canola or olive oil; 1–2 slices sprouted wheat toast with butter and an apple or pear.	One whole wheat tortilla spread with nut butter and apple butter and rolled up; handful of crudités with hummus dip, fruit.	Lamb chops or roast with rosemary (4–6 oz); sweet potato with onions carmelized in olive oil; leafy salad (2–3 cups) flaxseed oil & lemon juice dressing.
2	$^1/_2$–1 cup cooked barley with 1 cup frozen berries, partially thawed, and 1 tablespoon crispy nuts; stir in 1–2 tablespoons protein powder; may moisten with nut milk, coconut milk, rice milk.	Breakfast for lunch: Scrambled egg burritos with salsa, avocado, sprouts in corn tortillas; crudités and fruit.	Roast chicken; celery root purée; Swiss chard sautéed with garlic; fresh pineapple lightly broiled or grilled for dessert.
3	Lunch for breakfast: one slice dark dense bread or half a wholegrain bagel; 4 oz. chicken, lean beef or pork; lettuce and tomato/cucumber/radish/pepper/grated carrot/etc.	Crudités with chicken salad dip ($^1/_2$ cup); nut rice crackers; fruit.	White fish cooked in parchment-lined foil with scallions and cracked black pepper (4–6 oz.); wild/brown rice pilaf*; tossed salad; partially thawed frozen strawberries and frozen acai whirled in food processor until smooth for dessert.
4	$^1/_2$–1 cup cooked millet with $^1/_4$ cup coconut (unsweetened); 2–3 tablespoons crispy nuts; may moisten as above; stir in 1–2 tablespoons protein powder.	Fish salad (capers, diced tomatoes, and peppers mixed with olive oil/lemon juice and lightly tossed with leftover fish); serve on brown rice cakes or lettuce leaves; fruit for dessert.	Large salad (2–3 cups greens) with 4–6 oz. cooked shrimp or chicken; any veggies may be added; dressing: 1–2 tablespoons olive and flaxseed oils with vinegar or lemon juice, herbs, salt, and pepper; baked apple for dessert

*See recipe section.

Day	Breakfast	Lunch	Dinner
5	Smoothie: ¹/₂ cup nut milk or coconut milk or rice milk, ¹/₂ cup frozen berries, 2 tablespoons protein powder, 1 teaspoon honey; 2–3 tablespoons sheep milk yogurt for dessert.	¹/₄ pound burger (veggie, lean beef, buffalo, lamb, chicken, salmon) on tortilla (whole wheat, corn, rice flour); tomato, avocado, lettuce, sprouts, as you wish; season with mustard, low-sugar catsup; add fruit and crispy beans.	Grilled salmon; cabbage and red pepper slaw; new potatoes with arugula; lemon sorbet for dessert.
6	Salmon and Spinach frittata*; crudités.	One slice dark dense bread or half a wholegrain bagel; 4 oz. chicken, lean beef, or pork; lettuce and tomato/cucumber/radish/pepper/grated carrot/etc.; apple or pear.	Pork loin roast marinated in garlic-ginger-soy-vinegar; quinoa and butternut squash*; steamed beet greens with grated beets with olive oil and walnuts; raspberries and cashew cream for dessert.
7	Leftover dinner for breakfast: Have some of the meat and veggies from one of the previous nights.	Half an avocado filled with 3–4 oz. tiny canned shrimp mixed with lemon juice and canola mayo; Finn crisp crackers; fruit.	You can cheat on one meal a week and still be 95 percent compliant with the plan! (Cordain, *The Dietary Acne Cure*, 2007)

*See recipe section.

  lamb

  buffalo

  chicken

  turkey

  game meat

  eggs, especially omega-3 rich

  beans/tofu/tempe

  milk (also carbohydrate)

  cheese**

    sheep's milk—manchego (a mild hard cheese), Bulgarian sheep
    feta

    goat milk—soft cheeses, goat gouda (Cabanca, Arina), goat feta

  yogurt**

sheep's milk—Old Chatham Sheepherding Company

goat milk

nuts (also carbohydrate), raw & organic
    walnuts, almonds, hazelnuts, pecans, macadamia nuts, Brazil nuts,
    cashews

**Milk products may worsen acne in some people. Consider avoiding
these for one month. If your acne improves, consider non-cow dairy,
such as sheep or goat cheeses and yogurts. You may find that you
tolerate small amounts of cow dairy or only lactofermented cow dairy
(yogurt or kefir).*

CARBOHYDRATES

vegetable carbs

squash, winter

beans, dried and green
    canned white, black, chickpeas, black-eyed peas, kidney, lentils

sweet potatoes

white poatoes

peas

corn

whole grains

bulgar wheat

brown rice (try basmati brown)

wild rice

buckwheat groats (kasha)

quinoa

barley

oats, steel cut

millet

LEGUMES

lentils

dried beans and peas

BREADS AND PASTAS

whole grain (and sprouted, if possible)

ezekiel

wheat and corn tortillas

crackers/chips

whole grain crackers
    rye
    Finn Crisp
    Wasa

brown rice

wheat

Ak Mak

nut rice crackers

baked chips (potato, corn, rice)

FATS AND OILS

olive oil, extra virgin, organic

canola oil, cold pressed

flaxseed oil, cold pressed, dark container

butter

sesame oil, cold pressed

walnut oil, cold pressed

canola mayonnaise

Keep all oils, except olive oil, in the fridge or the freezer.

CONDIMENTS/SPICES/HERBS

mustard

catsup, low sugar

soy sauce

vinegar, unfiltered, raw, cider vinegar

rice vinegar

wine vinegar

salsa

bean dips

tapenade

pesto

hummus

ginger

rosemary

oregano

nutmeg

turmeric

cumin
dill
cilantro
basil

MISCELLANEOUS
rice protein powder or hemp protein powder
non-dairy milks: nut, rice, coconut
honey
stevia
salt
pepper
sherry

✖ ✖ ✖

We are deeply grateful to nutrition and culinary expert Dr. Gabriella Chow of Toronto for allowing us to present her special recipes as part of the Clear Skin Diet. (For more information, please visit www.gchownd.com.)

Tofu and Tempeh Dishes

SWISS CHARD WITH TOFU AND EDAMAME

SERVES 4

$\frac{1}{2}$ 454-gram package medium-firm tofu, drained and cut into cubes

2 tablespoons light soy sauce

2 teaspoons minced ginger root

2 cloves of garlic, crushed and minced

1 tablespoon cold-pressed, extra-virgin olive oil or organic canola oil

$1\frac{1}{2}$ cups sliced portabello mushrooms (or any other mushroom)

$\frac{2}{3}$ cup shelled edamame

$\frac{1}{2}$ teaspoon paprika

$\frac{1}{3}$ cup water

1   bunch Swiss chard, washed, stems and leaves torn into
     pieces
     Pepper to taste

1. Marinate cubed tofu in soy sauce for 5 minutes.

2. Sauté ginger and garlic in olive oil or canola oil for 1–2 minutes over
    medium heat.

3. Add mushrooms, edamame, and paprika. Sauté for another 2–3 min-
    utes.

4. Add $1/3$ cup water and Swiss chard in several small handfuls at a time
    to the skillet. Increase heat to boiling and cook 2–3 minutes or until all
    the Swiss chard is tender.

5. Season with pepper to taste.

SPICED CHICKPEAS AND TOFU

SERVES 4

1   small onion, diced
1   clove garlic, crushed and minced
1   tablespoon cold-pressed, extra-virgin olive oil or organic
     canola oil
2   cups sliced cremini (brown) mushrooms
2   teaspoons ground cumin
$1/2$ teaspoon turmeric
$1/4$ teaspoon black pepper
1   454-gram package medium-firm tofu, drained and cut
     into cubes
2   cups chickpeas (garbanzo beans), cooked or canned
     Salt to taste

1. Sauté onions and garlic in olive oil or canola oil for 1–2 minutes over
    medium heat.

2. Add mushrooms and sauté for another 2 minutes.

3. Stir in cumin, turmeric, black pepper, and tofu. Cook for another 2
    minutes.

4. Add chickpeas and salt to taste. Simmer for another 2 minutes.

SPINACH AND TOFU

SERVES 4

 $^{1}/_{2}$ cup water
 1   tablespoon cold-pressed, extra-virgin olive oil or organic
     canola oil
 1   cup chopped fresh cilantro (coriander) leaves
 1   teaspoon turmeric
 1   cup water
 1   10-ounce package fresh spinach
 1   454-gram package medium-firm tofu, drained and cut
     into cubes
 2   tablespoons soy sauce

1. Heat $^{1}/_{2}$ cup water to a boil over high heat. Add oil, cilantro, and tur-meric and reduce to medium heat. Cook for 1–2 minutes.

2. Add remaining ingredients, bring to a boil, then reduce heat to medium-low for 6 minutes, until spinach and tofu are cooked.

STIR-FRIED VEGETABLES AND TOFU

SERVES 6

 2   cups boiling water
 6   dried shiitake mushrooms, stems removed
 1   454-gram package soft tofu, drained and cut into cubes
 2   teaspoons soy sauce
 2   tablespoons cold-pressed, extra-virgin olive oil or organic
     canola oil
 $^{1}/_{2}$ onion, diced
 1   clove garlic, crushed and minced
 $^{1}/_{2}$ cup water
 4   stalks celery, diced
 2   carrots, diced
 2   cups green beans
 2   teaspoons salt
 $^{1}/_{4}$ teaspoon pepper
 $^{1}/_{4}$ cup finely chopped fresh cilantro (coriander) leaves

1. Pour 2 cups boiling water over dried shiitake mushrooms and allow to soften for about 1 hour. Slice mushrooms and reserve the mushroom liquid.

2. Marinate cubed tofu in 1^1/$_2$ cups of the mushroom liquid and 1 tea-spoon soy sauce for 20 minutes. Reserve ^{1}/$_2$ cup of the remaining mushroom liquid for the vegetables.

3. Sauté the onion and garlic in olive oil or canola oil for 1–2 minutes over medium heat.

4. Add ^{1}/$_2$ cup water and ^{1}/$_2$ cup of the reserved mushroom liquid and stir in sliced mushrooms, vegetables (celery, carrots, and green beans), salt, and pepper. Bring to a boil over high heat, then reduce to medium heat, cover, and cook for 5 minutes.

5. Add tofu (without the liquid it was marinating in), cilantro, and the remaining 1 teaspoon soy sauce. Turn down heat and simmer for 2 minutes.

6. Remove from heat and enjoy.

TEMPEH STIR-FRY

SERVES 4

1	250-gram package of tempeh, torn into bite-size pieces
2	tablespoons cold-pressed, extra-virgin olive oil or organic canola oil
2	tablespoons dark soy sauce
1	tablespoon lime juice
1	red bell pepper, diced
1	8-ounce (250 g) package cremini (brown) mushrooms, sliced
^{1}/$_2$	of a 10-ounce package fresh spinach (5 ounces)

1. Sauté tempeh in oil, soy sauce, and lime juice over medium heat for 1 minute.

2. Stir in bell pepper, mushrooms, and spinach and cook for 3–4 minutes until vegetables have cooked through and are tender.

TEMPEH QUINOA SALAD

SERVES 4

2	cups water
1	cup quinoa, uncooked
1/2	250-gram package of tempeh, torn into bite-sized pieces
2/3	cup soy mayonnaise (e.g., Nasoya Nayonaise sandwich spread)
1 1/2	tablespoons soy sauce
2	stalks celery, finely diced
3	green onions, finely chopped

1. Bring 2 cups water to a boil, add quinoa, bring back to a boil, then reduce heat to medium, cover and cook for 10–12 minutes (until the quinoa has soaked up all the water).

2. While the quinoa is cooking, place a metal colander in the same pot over the quinoa and steam the tempeh, with the pot covered.

3. In a medium bowl, mix the soy mayonnaise, soy sauce, celery, and onions to make the dressing.

4. When the quinoa and tempeh have finished cooking, mix the dressing with the quinoa and tempeh until well combined.

Soups

CARROT AND GINGER SOUP

SERVES 6

3	teaspoons minced ginger root
1	clove garlic, crushed and minced
1	tablespoon cold-pressed, extra-virgin olive oil or organic canola oil
1	cup water
6	medium carrots, peeled and thinly sliced
1	teaspoon salt
3	cups vanilla rice milk (e.g., Rice Dream)

1. Sauté 1 teaspoon ginger root and 1 clove minced garlic in olive oil or canola oil for 1–2 minutes over medium heat.

2. Add water, carrots, and 1 teaspoon of ginger root, bring to a boil, then reduce to moderate heat and cover. Remove from heat when carrots are tender (about 10 minutes).

3. In 2 or 3 separate batches, pour carrots and vanilla rice milk into a blender and puree. *Be careful to start the blender on low speed so the hot soup does not erupt and burn you. And make sure you don't fill the blender more than half full.*

4. Pour the puréed liquid back into the pot over low heat to keep warm and add the remaining 1 teaspoon minced ginger root.

5. If the soup is too thick, stir in 1 cup (more or less, depending on how thick or thin you want the soup) boiling water.

MISO TOFU SOUP

SERVES 6

    6   green onions, finely chopped
    2   tablespoons cold-pressed, extra-virgin olive oil or organic
         canola oil
    5½ cups water
    ⅓   of a 454-gram package soft tofu, drained and cut into
         small cubes
    ⅓   cup white miso

1. Sauté green onions in olive oil or canola oil for 1–2 minutes over medium heat.

2. Add water and tofu to green onions.

3. In a small bowl, add enough boiling water to miso, stirring until miso dissolves and is smooth. Add to pot.

4. Heat soup for several minutes while gently stirring to mix all ingredients, but do not boil. (If the soup is too salty for your taste, add more water, if it is not salty enough, add more miso.)

SPLIT PEA AND VEGETABLE SOUP

SERVES 4

1	small onion, diced
1	tablespoon cold-pressed, extra-virgin olive oil or organic canola oil
1	carrot, diced finely
1	stalk celery, diced finely
4	cups water
1	cup yellow split peas
1	teaspoon salt
2	bay leaves
1	teaspoon finely chopped fresh rosemary leaves

1. Sauté onion in olive oil or canola oil for 1–2 minutes over medium heat.

2. Add carrots and celery and sauté for another 2–3 minutes over medium heat.

3. Add remaining ingredients. Bring to a boil, then reduce to a simmer and cover, cooking until split peas are tender, about 45–50 minutes.

4. Remove bay leaves before eating.

LENTIL, BARLEY, AND VEGETABLE SOUP

SERVES 6

1	onion, diced
2	cloves garlic, crushed and minced
1	tablespoon cold-pressed, extra-virgin olive oil or organic canola oil
2	carrots, diced
2	stalks celery, diced
1 1/2	teaspoons dried thyme
6	cups water
1/2	cup dried lentils
1/3	cup pot barley, soaked 4 hours or overnight in water
2	bay leaves
1	sweet potato, peeled and diced
2	cups broccoli florets
1/4	cup finely chopped fresh flat-leaf parsley leaves
	Salt and pepper to taste

1. Sauté onion and garlic in olive oil or canola oil for 1–2 minutes over medium heat.

2. Add carrots, celery, and thyme and sauté for another 3 minutes until softened.

3. Add water then lentils, barley, and bay leaves. Bring to a boil, reduce heat to low and simmer, covered, for 45 minutes.

4. Add sweet potato and broccoli and simmer about 20 minutes more or until potato and barley are tender.

5. Remove bay leaves and stir in parsley.

6. Add salt and pepper to taste.

MULTI-GREENS SOUP

SERVES 6

1	leek (white part only), sliced
2	cups sliced zucchini
2	cups broccoli florets
2	cloves garlic, crushed and minced
1	teaspoon dried thyme
1	bay leaf
1	teaspoon salt
4	cups water
1½	cups vanilla rice milk (e.g., Rice Dream)
	Pepper to taste

1. In a large pot, combine all the ingredients except the rice milk and pepper (leek, zucchini, broccoli, garlic, thyme, bay leaf, salt, and water). Bring to a boil, then reduce to a simmer and cover. Remove from heat when vegetables are tender (about 10 minutes).

2. Remove the bay leaf, and in three separate batches, pour vegetables and the water it was cooking in into a blender and puree. *Be careful to start the blender on low speed so the hot soup does not erupt and burn you. And make sure you don't fill the blender more than half full.*

3. Pour puréed liquid back into pot over low heat to keep warm and add vanilla rice milk and pepper to taste. Stir to mix thoroughly and enjoy.

CREAMY CAULIFLOWER AND SWEET POTATO SOUP

SERVES 6

3	cloves garlic, crushed and minced
2	tablespoons cold-pressed, extra-virgin olive oil or organic canola oil
1	tablespoon water
1	teaspoon ground cumin
4	cups water
1	small cauliflower, cut into florets
1	large sweet potato, peeled and cut into bite-size cubes
1	cup vanilla rice milk (e.g., Rice Dream)
2	teaspoons dried basil
	Salt to taste

1. Sauté minced garlic in olive oil or canola oil for 1–2 minutes over medium heat.

2. Add 1 tablespoon water and ground cumin (add more water if necessary to prevent the cumin from sticking to the pan) and cook over medium heat for 1 minute.

3. Add water, cauliflower, and sweet potato. Bring to a boil, then reduce to moderate heat and cover. Remove from heat when vegetables are tender (about 20 minutes).

4. Set aside 2 cups cooked vegetables. In two or three separate batches, pour cooked vegetables and vanilla rice milk into a blender and puree. *Be careful to start the blender on low speed so the hot soup does not erupt and burn you. And make sure you don't fill the blender more than half full.*

5. Pour puréed liquid back into pot with the reserved vegetables over low heat to keep warm and add dried basil and salt to taste.

Vegetable Dishes

HERB AND MUSHROOM SWEET POTATO SIDE

SERVES 6

2	large (or 3 medium) sweet potatoes
$\frac{1}{2}$	onion, diced
1	clove garlic, crushed and minced
2	tablespoons cold-pressed, extra-virgin olive oil or organic canola oil
1	8-ounce (250 g) package cremini (brown) mushrooms, thinly sliced and diced into small pieces
$\frac{1}{4}$	cup finely chopped fresh cilantro (coriander) leaves
$\frac{1}{2}$	teaspoon dried thyme
$\frac{3}{4}$	cup vanilla rice milk (e.g., Rice Dream)
	Salt and pepper to taste

1. Scrub potatoes to clean. Place in pot with just enough water to cover the bottom half of the potatoes. Cover, bring to a boil, and simmer until tender, 20–30 minutes.

2. Meanwhile, sauté onions and garlic in olive oil or canola oil for 1–2 minutes over medium heat. Add mushrooms, cilantro, and thyme and cook for another 2 minutes.

3. Add rice milk. Bring to a boil, then reduce to a simmer to keep warm.

4. When potatoes are tender and thoroughly cooked, drain and pat dry.

5. Cut into and remove a portion of sweet potato, add in mushroom mixture.

6. Season to taste with salt and pepper.

HONEY-AND-BALSAMIC-GLAZED BEETS AND CARROTS

SERVES **4** TO **6**

- ¹/₂ cup water
- 2   tablespoons honey
- 1   tablespoon balsamic vinegar
- 3   medium beets, peeled and sliced
- 3   medium carrots, peeled and sliced
- 2   teaspoons finely minced fresh thyme

1. Heat water until it boils and add honey, balsamic vinegar, beets, and carrots. Reduce heat to a simmer, cover, and allow to simmer for about 25–30 minutes or until vegetables are tender and most of the liquid has been absorbed.

2. Toward the end of the cooking time, add thyme.

PORTABELLO MUSHROOMS, BEETS, AND TURNIPS SAUTÉED IN BALSAMIC VINEGAR

Serves 4

- 4   tablespoons water
- 2   tablespoons cold-pressed, extra-virgin olive oil or organic canola oil
- 1¹/₂ teaspoons balsamic vinegar
- 2   teaspoons soy sauce
- 2   turnips, peeled and sliced into ¹/₂-inch rectangular slices
- 1   beet, peeled and sliced into ¹/₂-inch rectangular slices
- 2   portabello mushroom caps, sliced

1. Combine water, oil, balsamic vinegar, and soy sauce and bring to a boil over medium-high heat. Add beets and turnips. Reduce heat to a simmer, cover, and allow to simmer for about 10 minutes.

2. Add mushroom caps, cover, and allow to simmer for another 5 minutes or until vegetables are tender and most of the liquid has been absorbed.

SESAME-GLAZED CARROT AND BURDOCK SAUTÉ

SERVES 4

1	tablespoon sesame oil
2	burdock roots (gobo), each about 12 inches long, sliced into matchstick-size pieces (julienned)*
1	cup water
1	large carrot, sliced into matchstick-sized pieces (julienned)
1	tablespoon soy sauce
$\frac{1}{2}$	teaspoon salt

1. Sauté burdock in sesame oil for 2–3 minutes over medium heat.

2. Add $\frac{1}{2}$ cup water, bring to a boil, cover, and continue to cook over medium heat for 5 minutes.

3. Add carrots, soy sauce, salt, and remaining $\frac{1}{2}$ cup water. Bring to a boil, cover, and continue to cook over medium heat for another 5 minutes until vegetables are tender.

   *Prepare burdock by washing the burdock and scraping the outer skin lightly with a sharp knife. The skin does not need to be peeled, as most of the nutrients are found in the skin. The julienned slices should immediately be submerged in salted cold water to prevent them from discoloring (which occurs quickly) and to moderate the strong taste (which can overpower a recipe).

Grain Dishes

BROWN RICE WITH KALE AND TOMATOES

SERVES 4 TO 6

1	cup brown rice, uncooked
2	cups water
1	clove garlic, crushed and minced
1	tablespoon cold-pressed, extra-virgin olive oil or organic canola oil
2	large tomatoes, diced
2½	cups finely chopped kale leaves, stems removed
1	teaspoon salt

1. Bring 2 cups of water to a boil. Add 1 cup brown rice. Cover pan, lower heat, and simmer for about 50 minutes. When all the water has been absorbed and rice is cooked, toss rice with a fork and let stand for a few minutes.

2. Sauté garlic in olive oil or canola oil for 1–2 minutes over medium heat.

3. Add tomatoes, kale, and salt and cook over medium heat for 4 minutes.

4. In a large bowl, combine the kale and tomato mixture with brown rice.

OKRA AND BROWN RICE WITH SALMON

SERVES 4

3	tablespoons water
2	tablespoons cold-pressed, extra-virgin olive oil or organic canola oil
1	tablespoon tomato paste
12	small pieces fresh okra
1	teaspoon salt
2	cups water
1	cup brown rice, uncooked
1	teaspoon dried basil
2	cans wild Pacific salmon
1	large tomato, diced

1. In a pot, heat water, oil, and tomato paste over medium heat.

2. Add okra and salt and sauté for 3 minutes.

3. Add water and brown rice and bring to a boil. Cover pot, lower heat, and simmer for about 50 minutes. In the last 5 minutes of cooking,

add basil and remove bones from salmon, flake the fish meat with a fork, and add to pot with rice.

4. When all the water has been absorbed and rice is cooked, add diced tomato and mix well.

PINEAPPLE-TOFU FRIED RICE

SERVES 4

1	cup brown rice, uncooked
2	cups water
1	454-gram package medium-firm tofu, drained and cut into cubes
1	tablespoon soy sauce
2	tablespoons cooking sherry
2	cloves garlic, crushed and minced
1	tablespoon minced ginger root
2	tablespoons cold pressed, extra-virgin olive oil or organic canola oil
$1/_3$	cup pineapple juice
1	cup each finely diced carrots and frozen peas (or 2 cups frozen mixed vegetables)
$1/_2$	teaspoon salt
1	cup small-bite-size chunks fresh pineapple

1. Bring 2 cups water to a boil. Add 1 cup brown rice. Cover pan, lower heat, and simmer for about 50 minutes. When all the water has been absorbed and rice is cooked, toss rice with a fork and let stand for a few minutes.

2. Place cubed tofu in a large bowl. Combine soy sauce and cooking sherry and pour over tofu. Marinate for 1 hour.

3. When rice is cooked, sauté garlic and ginger root in olive oil or canola oil for 1–2 minutes over medium heat.

4. Add pineapple juice, 1 cup carrots and 1 cup frozen peas (or 2 cups frozen mixed vegetables), and salt and sauté for another 4–5 minutes or until vegetables are tender. (If using frozen vegetables, sauté for only 2–3 minutes.)

5. Add brown rice, tofu and the liquid it was marinating in, and pineapple to skillet and cook until rice and tofu are heated through (another 1–2 minutes).

QUINOA AND BUTTERNUT SQUASH

SERVES 4

    1   cup water

    1   tablespoon cold-pressed, extra-virgin olive oil or organic canola oil

    3¹/₂   cups bite-size cubes of peeled butternut squash

    ¹/₄   cup finely chopped fresh cilantro (coriander) leaves

    2   cups water

    1   cup quinoa, uncooked

    1   teaspoon white miso

1. Bring 1 cup water to a boil, add oil and butternut squash, bring back to a boil, then reduce heat to medium and cook until squash is tender, about 15–20 minutes. Toward the end of cooking, add the chopped cilantro leaves.

2. While squash is cooking, bring 2 cups water to a boil, add quinoa, bring back to a boil, then reduce heat to medium, cover, and cook for 10–12 minutes (until the quinoa has soaked up all the water).

3. When both squash and quinoa have finished cooking, carefully mix them together in a large bowl without breaking up the squash.

4. Dissolve miso in a small amount of hot water and stir into the squash mixture.

MILLET PILAF WITH CARROTS AND PEAS

SERVES 4

    1   cup millet

    1   small onion, diced

    1   clove garlic, crushed and minced

    1   tablespoon cold-pressed, extra-virgin olive oil or organic canola oil

    1   cup water

    ¹/₂   cup vanilla rice milk (e.g., Rice Dream)

    2   cups grated (shredded) carrots

    1   teaspoon salt

    1   cup frozen peas

    1   teaspoon dried basil

1. In a heavy pan over medium heat, toast millet, stirring constantly, until you hear the seeds pop and the seeds are fragrant, about 3–4 minutes. Set aside in a bowl.

2. Sauté onion and garlic in olive oil or canola oil for 1–2 minutes over medium heat.

3. Add water, rice milk, and millet. Stir well so that all the millet is coated. Add carrots on top of millet mixture and sprinkle with salt. Bring to a boil and reduce to medium-low heat. Cover and cook until liquid is absorbed, about 20–25 minutes. Note: Add frozen peas on top of carrots halfway through cooking.

4. When all the liquid is absorbed and millet is cooked, remove from heat, add basil, and mix well with a fork.

MILLET AND CAULIFLOWER IN MISO SAUCE

SERVES 6

2	cloves garlic, crushed and minced
1	tablespoon cold-pressed, extra-virgin olive oil or organic canola oil
2½	cups water
1	cup millet
½	medium-sized cauliflower, stems and florets sliced thinly
3	green onions, finely chopped
½	teaspoon salt
½	cup boiling water
1	tablespoon white miso

1. Sauté garlic in olive oil or canola oil for 1–2 minutes over medium heat.

2. Add water, millet, cauliflower, green onions, and salt. Bring to a boil then reduce to a simmer. Cover and cook until liquid is absorbed, about 20 minutes.

3. When all the liquid is absorbed and millet is cooked, remove from heat. Dissolve miso in boiling water and add to millet mixture, mixing well.

WILD/BROWN RICE PILAF

Serves 6

2	cloves garlic, crushed and minced
1	tablespoon minced ginger root
2	tablespoons cold-pressed, extra-virgin olive oil or organic canola oil
1	leek, including both white and green parts, sliced
1	bunch asparagus, sliced into 1/2-inch bite-size pieces
6	stalks celery, diced
4	oyster mushrooms, sliced (or any other mushrooms)
1	cup water
2	teaspoons salt
1/4	teaspoon pepper
3	cups steamed wild or brown rice (see below)
2	tablespoons soy sauce
1/2	cup finely chopped fresh cilantro (coriander) leaves

1. In a large pot, sauté garlic and ginger in olive oil or canola oil for 1–2 minutes over medium heat.

2. Add leek and sauté until it softens, about 4 minutes.

3. Add asparagus, celery, mushrooms, water, salt, and pepper. Bring to a boil on high heat, then reduce to medium heat, cover and cook for 5 minutes.

4. Add rice, soy sauce, cilantro, and stir to blend. Cover and simmer for 3 minutes.

5. Remove from heat, serve using a pasta spoon to strain out any extra liquid, and enjoy.

WILD RICE

Makes 3 cups steamed wild rice

Rinse 1 cup wild rice. Place in pot with 3 cups water and 1/4 teaspoon salt. Bring to a boil, cover, and reduce heat to a simmer for 1 hour or until the grains are soft and the water is absorbed. Remove from heat and allow to steam, covered, for 5–10 minutes. Fluff with a fork.

WILD RICE, BARLEY, AND CHICKPEA SALAD

SERVES 6

> 4 cups water
>
> 2 teaspoons salt
>
> $1/2$ cup pot barley, soaked for 4 hours or overnight (grain becomes softer and more tender)
>
> $1/2$ cup wild rice
>
> $2^1/2$ cups chickpeas (garbanzo beans), cooked or canned
>
> $1/4$ cup cold-pressed, extra-virgin olive oil

1. Bring water to a boil in a large pot.

2. Add 1 teaspoon salt, barley, and wild rice. Cover, reduce heat to a simmer, and cook for 60–70 minutes without stirring or lifting the lid.

3. When the barley and wild rice are soft and tender, strain out any remaining liquid and mix well with chickpeas, 1 teaspoon salt, and olive oil.

Bean Dishes

KIDNEY BEAN AND BUTTERNUT SQUASH STEW

SERVES 6

6	cups water
2	cups dried red kidney beans, soaked overnight (at least 8 hours) (or 4–5 cups of canned red kidney beans)
2	bay leaves
3	cloves garlic, crushed and minced
1	tablespoon cold-pressed, extra-virgin olive oil or organic canola oil
1	cup water
4^1/$_2$	cups cubed, bite-size pieces of peeled butternut squash
3	tomatoes, diced
^{1}/$_2$	cup chopped flat-leaf parsley leaves
2	teaspoons dried basil
	Salt

1. Bring 6 cups water to a boil in a large pot. Add beans and bay leaves. Bring back to a boil, then reduce to medium heat and cook, partially covered, until beans are tender, about 90 minutes.

2. Meanwhile, in another pan sauté the garlic in olive oil or canola oil for 1–2 minutes over medium heat.

3. Add 1 cup water and squash, bring to a boil, then reduce to medium heat, cover, and cook until squash is tender, about 20 minutes. Toward the end of cooking, add tomatoes, parsley, basil, and salt.

4. When beans have finished cooking, remove bay leaves and mix squash mixture into beans, adding more salt to taste if desired.

BLACK BEANS AND TEMPEH

SERVES 4

2	cloves garlic, crushed and minced
1	tablespoon cold-pressed, extra-virgin olive oil or organic canola oil
1	red bell pepper, diced
1	stalk celery, diced
2	cups cooked/canned black beans
1	cup frozen corn
^{1}/$_2$	of a 250-gram package tempeh, torn into bite-size pieces

2 tablespoons tomato paste

1 tablespoon lime juice

$^1/_2$ cup finely chopped fresh cilantro (coriander) leaves

1 teaspoon dried oregano

$^1/_2$ teaspoon salt

$^1/_2$ teaspoon pepper

1. Sauté garlic in olive oil or canola oil for 1–2 minutes over medium heat.

2. Add bell pepper and celery and sauté for another 3–4 minutes over medium heat until vegetables are tender.

3. Add the remaining ingredients, mix well, increase heat to medium-high, and cook for another 3 minutes.

CARROTS AND LENTILS

SERVES 4 TO 6

$^1/_2$ onion, diced

2 cloves garlic, crushed and minced

2 tablespoons cold-pressed, extra-virgin olive oil or organic canola oil

1 large carrot, diced

1 teaspoon dried thyme

2$^1/_2$ cups water

1 cup dried lentils

1 bay leaf

1 teaspoon salt

$^1/_4$ teaspoon pepper

1. Sauté onion and garlic in olive oil or canola oil for 1–2 minutes over medium heat.

2. Add carrots and thyme and sauté for another 1–2 minutes.

3. Add water, lentils, bay leaf, salt, and pepper. Bring to a boil over high heat, then reduce to medium-low heat and simmer, partially covered, until lentils are just tender and most of the water has been absorbed, about 30 minutes.

4. Remove bay leaf and add more salt and pepper if desired.

Salads

SPINACH AND BERRY SALAD

SERVES 6

Dressing:

1/2   cup cold-pressed, extra-virgin olive oil or organic canola oil

1/4   cup white wine vinegar

1/4   teaspoon paprika

3   tablespoons sugar

6   cups bite-size pieces fresh spinach, washed, and dried

1   pint fresh strawberries, stems removed and sliced

1/2   cup fresh blueberries

1/2   cup pine nuts

1.   Mix together all the ingredients for the salad dressing.

2.   Toss well with all other ingredients, and let marinate for at least 15 minutes before serving.

BEET, PEAR, AND CRANBERRY SALAD

SERVES 6

3   beets, peeled and cubed into bite-size pieces

2/3   cup peach jam

1   tablespoon lime juice

2   teaspoons dijon mustard

4   Bartlett pears, peeled and cubed into bite-sized pieces

1   cup dried cranberries (You may soak them in water for 5–10 minutes if you prefer your cranberries soft and plump.)

1.   Steam cubed beets in a colander until tender, about 20 minutes. Set aside to cool.

2.   In a small saucepan, heat jam, lime juice, and Dijon mustard over low heat and stir until blended.

3.   In a large bowl, mix together the beets, pears, cranberries, and warm peach sauce. Toss well to coat.

QUINOA SALAD WITH MANGO

SERVES 6

2	cups water
1	cup quinoa, uncooked
$^2/_3$	cup soy mayonnaise (e.g., Nasoya Nayonaise sandwich spread)
$^1/_2$	cup finely chopped fresh dill, stems removed
1	teaspoon paprika
1	large tomato, diced
2	red peppers, diced
1	large cucumber, peeled and diced
2	ripe mangoes, peeled, seeded, and diced
$^1/_2$	teaspoon salt (or more to taste)

1. Bring 2 cups water to a boil, add quinoa, bring back to a boil, then reduce heat to medium, cover and cook for 10–12 minutes (until the quinoa has soaked up all the water). Set aside and allow to cool.

2. In a medium bowl, mix the soy mayonnaise, dill, and paprika to make the dressing.

3. In a large bowl, mix the quinoa with the diced tomatoes, red peppers, cucumber, mangoes, dressing, and salt until well combined.

BRUSSELS SPROUT SALAD

SERVES 4 TO 6

4	cups halved Brussels sprouts
$^3/_4$	cup thinly-sliced sun-dried tomato halves in oil
1	cup cherry tomatoes
$^1/_2$	cup white wine vinegar
$^1/_2$	cup cold-pressed, extra-virgin olive oil or organic canola oil
4	green onions, finely chopped

1. Boil halved Brussels sprouts in salted water until just tender (this should take no more than 10 minutes). Drain and put in a large salad bowl.

2. Toss well with all other ingredients and serve chilled.

Omega-3 Fish Dishes

SALMON DILL SOUP

SERVES 4 TO 6

  2   medium salmon fillets, skin removed (about ³/₄ pound total)

  2   cups water

  1   medium sweet potato, peeled and diced into bite-size pieces

  2   medium carrots, peeled and diced into bite-size pieces

  ¹/₂ onion, diced

  3   cups vanilla rice milk (e.g., Rice Dream)

  ¹/₂ cup finely chopped fresh dill, stems removed

  1   teaspoon salt

  6   tablespoons cornstarch

1. Slice each salmon fillet very thinly into bite-size pieces. Set aside.

2. In a pot, bring water, sweet potato, carrots, and onion to a boil, then reduce to medium-high heat, cover, and cook until vegetables are tender, about 10 minutes.

3. Add rice milk and bring to a boil.

4. Add salmon, dill, and salt, and reduce heat to medium until salmon is done, about 3 minutes.

5. Mix cornstarch with just enough cold water to dissolve and add to soup. Bring soup to a boil while stirring, and allow mixture to thicken for 1–2 minutes.

6. Remove from heat and serve warm.

SALMON CORN CHOWDER

SERVES 4 TO 6

2	medium salmon fillets, skin removed (about ¾ pound total)
½	onion, diced
2	tablespoons cold-pressed, extra-virgin olive oil or organic canola oil
½	cup diced red bell pepper
½	cup diced celery
4	cups vegetable stock, salt-reduced
2	cups frozen corn
3	tablespoons flour
⅔	cup finely chopped fresh flat-leaf parsley leaves

1. Slice each salmon fillet very thinly into bite-size pieces. Set aside.

2. In a pot, sauté onion in olive oil or canola oil for 1–2 minutes over medium heat.

3. Add red bell pepper and celery and continue to sauté for another 4 minutes over medium heat or until vegetables are tender.

4. Add vegetable stock, corn, and flour and continue to cook for another 4 minutes over medium heat or until mixture thickens slightly.

5. Stir in sliced salmon pieces and flat-leaf parsley and cook for another 3 minutes until salmon is cooked through.

SALMON FETTUCCINE WITH SWISS CHARD IN TOMATO SAUCE

SERVES 6

6	cups water
1	340-gram package whole wheat fettuccine pasta, dried (or any other type of pasta)
1	tablespoon salt
2	medium salmon fillets, skin removed (about ³/₄ pound total)
3	cloves garlic, crushed and minced
2	tablespoons cold-pressed, extra-virgin olive oil or organic canola oil
3	cups tomato sauce
2	cups thinly sliced cremini (brown) mushrooms
6	cups washed and thinly sliced Swiss chard (stems and leaves)
	Dried basil to taste

1. Bring water to a boil and add pasta and salt. Cook, uncovered, stirring occasionally until desired tenderness, about 15–20 minutes. Drain well.

2. While pasta is cooking, slice each salmon fillet into several thin pieces to ensure even cooking. Set aside.

3. In a skillet, sauté garlic in olive oil or canola oil for 1–2 minutes over medium heat.

4. Add tomato sauce, mushrooms, and Swiss chard and bring to a boil. Cover, decrease to medium heat, and cook until chard is tender, about 3–4 minutes.

5. Add salmon and bring back to a boil. Cover, decrease to medium heat, and cook for another 3 minutes until salmon is cooked through.

6. Add drained pasta to the salmon mixture, mix well, and add dried basil to taste.

TERIYAKI SALMON

SERVES 2

 2   medium salmon fillets, skin removed (about ³/₄ pound total)
 2   tablespoons water
 4   tablespoons teriyaki sauce
 1   tablespoon honey
 1   tablespoon cold-pressed, extra-virgin olive oil or organic canola oil

1. Slice each salmon fillet into several thin pieces to ensure even cooking.

2. In a skillet, heat water, teriyaki sauce, honey, and oil over high heat until boiling.

3. Add salmon, reduce to low heat, and cover.

4. Continue to cook over low heat until salmon is done, about 3–4 minutes.

MISO-AND-HERB SALMON

THIS IS A DELICIOUS SALMON RECIPE THAT IS QUICK AND EASY TO MAKE. SERVE IT OVER BROWN RICE AND ADD A SIDE OF VEGETABLES TO MAKE A COMPLETE AND HEALTHY MEAL. SERVES 2

 2   medium salmon fillets, skin removed (about ³/₄ pound total)
 2   teaspoons white miso
 ¹/₄ cup boiling water
 1   teaspoon finely chopped fresh basil
 1   teaspoon finely chopped fresh rosemary leaves

1. Slice each salmon fillet into several thin pieces to ensure even cooking.

2. Dissolve miso in boiling water and add herbs.

3. In a skillet, heat miso-herb mixture over high heat until boiling.

4. Add salmon, reduce to low heat, and cover.

5. Continue to cook over low heat until salmon is done, about 3–4 minutes.

ORANGE-AND-BALSAMIC SALMON

ANOTHER QUICK AND EASY SALMON RECIPE FOR THOSE WHO ENJOY THE TANG OF CITRUS WITH A TOUCH OF VINEGAR. SERVE IT OVER BROWN RICE AND ADD A SIDE OF VEGETABLES TO MAKE A COMPLETE AND HEALTHY MEAL. SERVES 2

2   medium salmon fillets, skin removed (about ¾ pound total)

1   small onion, diced 1   tablespoon cold-pressed, extra-virgin olive oil or organic canola oil

½   cup orange juice

1   tablespoon balsamic vinegar

3   teaspoons finely chopped fresh mint

3   teaspoons finely chopped fresh flat-leaf parsley leaves

Salt and pepper to taste

1. Slice each salmon fillet into several thin pieces to ensure even cooking.

2. Sauté onion in olive oil or canola oil for 1–2 minutes over medium heat.

3. In a small bowl, mix orange juice and balsamic vinegar. Add to sautéed onion. Increase heat to high until boiling.

4. Add salmon, herbs, and salt and pepper to taste, reduce to low heat, and cover.

5. Continue to cook over low heat until salmon is done, about 3–4 minutes.

HONEY-POACHED MACKEREL

SERVES 4

2	fresh whole mackerels
$^1/_2$	cup water
1	tablespoon soy sauce
2	tablespoons honey
2	teaspoons minced ginger root
2	green onions, finely chopped
2	tablespoons cornstarch

1. Cut the heads and tails off the mackerels. Wash and clean the fish with water. Slice fish lengthwise along the backbone so that half the fish is a fillet and the other half has the bone. Remove the bone. Slice each fillet in half again, resulting in 4 pieces per fish.

2. Combine water, soy sauce, honey, and ginger root in a bowl. Place the fish fillets in the bowl and marinate for 30 minutes.

3. Remove fish and heat the marinade over high heat. Bring to a boil.

4. Add fish (skin side down) and onions, cover, and reduce heat to a simmer. Continue to simmer until fish is done, about 3–4 minutes.

5. When fish is done, remove from heat, but leave the poaching liquid in the skillet.

6. In a small bowl, add just enough cold water to dissolve the cornstarch. Add the dissolved cornstarch to the poaching liquid and bring to a boil while stirring constantly. As soon as the liquid thickens and forms a thick sauce, remove from heat and drizzle over the fish before serving.

MAPLE-AND-SHERRY POACHED MACKEREL

SERVES 4

2	fresh whole mackerels
1/3	cup rice vinegar
1/4	cup soy sauce
1/4	cup cooking sherry
1/4	cup maple syrup
2	tablespoons cornstarch

1. Cut the heads and tails off the mackerels. Wash and clean the fish with water. Slice fish lengthwise along the backbone so that half the fish is a fillet and the other half has the bone. Remove the bone. Slice each fillet in half again, giving 4 pieces per fish.

2. Combine the rice vinegar, soy sauce, cooking sherry, and maple syrup in a bowl. Place the fish fillets in the bowl and marinate for 30 minutes.

3. Remove the fish and heat the marinade over high heat. Bring to a boil.

4. Add fish (skin side down), cover, and reduce heat to a simmer. Continue to simmer until fish is done, about 3–4 minutes.

5. When fish is done, remove from heat, but leave the poaching liquid in the skillet.

6. In a small bowl, add just enough cold water to dissolve the cornstarch. Add the dissolved cornstarch to the poaching liquid and bring to a boil while stirring constantly. As soon as the liquid thickens and forms a thick sauce, remove from heat and drizzle over the fish before serving.

MACKEREL-AND-SWEET-POTATO SALAD

SERVES 4

2	medium sweet potatoes
3	tablespoons cold-pressed, extra-virgin olive oil
1	tablespoon white wine vinegar
	Salt and pepper to taste
1/2	lemon
2	125-gram cans ready-to-eat mackerel fillets packed in water or brine
1	cup chopped tomatoes
1	tablespoon finely chopped fresh dill, stems removed

1. Scrub potatoes to clean. Place in pot with just enough water to cover

the bottom half of the potatoes. Cover, bring to a boil, and simmer until tender, 20–30 minutes.

2. Meanwhile, mix together the olive oil, vinegar, salt, pepper, and juice from ½ a lemon.

3. Reheat the mackerel, remove the skin, and flake the fish meat with a fork.

4. When potatoes are tender, remove from heat, drain, and pat dry. Remove peel. Cut potatoes into chunks.

5. In a large bowl, mix together the potatoes, flaked mackerel, tomatoes, dill, and dressing.

MACKEREL AND BROWN RICE

Serves 4

2	cups water
1	cup brown rice, uncooked
2	ready-to-eat mackerel fillets packed in water or brine
2	teaspoons Dijon mustard
1	tablespoon white wine vinegar
3	tablespoons cold-pressed, extra-virgin olive oil
	Pepper to taste

1. Bring 2 cups water to a boil. Add 1 cup brown rice. Cover pan, lower heat, and simmer about 50 minutes. When all the water has absorbed and rice is cooked, toss rice with a fork and let stand for a few minutes.

2. Reheat the mackerel, remove the skin, and flake the fish meat with a fork.

3. Whisk together the mustard, vinegar, and olive oil to make a dressing.

4. Mix together the rice, flaked mackerel, and dressing. Sprinkle with pepper to taste.

SARDINE SALAD

SERVES **6**

    1   cucumber, peeled and diced

    3   tomatoes, diced

    1   cup chopped flat-leaf parsley leaves

    4   cups mixed leafy greens

    2   cans sardines packed in water (8 sardines in total), bones removed

    $1/2$ cup cold-pressed, extra-virgin olive oil

    1   lemon

    1   tablespoon balsamic vinegar

    $1/2$ teaspoon dried basil

        Salt and pepper to taste

1. Combine cucumber, tomatoes, parsley leaves, and mixed leafy greens in a large bowl and toss to mix.

2. Remove fish from can and drain to remove water. In a small bowl, flake the fish meat with a fork.

3. In another bowl, whisk together oil, the juice of one lemon, balsamic vinegar, dried basil, and salt and pepper.

4. Add flaked fish meat and dressing to salad and toss well to combine.

SARDINE PASTA SALAD

SERVES **3** TO **4**

    3   cups water

    2   cups whole wheat fusilli pasta, dried

    1   teaspoon salt

    1   can sardines packed in water (4 sardines in total), bones removed

    1   tomato, diced

    $1/4$ cup finely chopped fresh cilantro (coriander) leaves

    3   tablespoons soy mayonnaise (e.g., Nasoya Nayonaise sandwich spread)

    $1/2$ teaspoon dried basil

        Salt and pepper to taste

1. Bring water to a boil and add pasta and salt. Cook, uncovered, stirring occasionally until desired tenderness, about 15–20 minutes. Drain well.

2. While pasta is cooking, remove fish from can and drain to remove water. In a small bowl, flake the fish meat with a fork.

3. Combine the remaining ingredients with the cooked pasta and flaked fish in a large bowl and toss to mix.

Omega-3 Egg Dishes

SALMON AND SPINACH FRITTATA

SERVES 6

2	cloves garlic, crushed and minced
2	tablespoons cold-pressed, extra-virgin olive oil or organic canola oil
1	cup thinly sliced cremini (brown) mushrooms
1/2	of a 10-ounce package fresh spinach
3/4	cups finely chopped green onions
1/2	teaspoon dried basil
1/4	teaspoon salt
1/4	teaspoon pepper
8	omega-3 eggs
1/4	cup vanilla rice milk (e.g., Rice Dream)
1	184-gram can boneless wild Pacific salmon, separated into chunks

1. In a skillet, sauté garlic in olive oil or canola oil for 1–2 minutes over medium heat.

2. Add mushrooms, spinach, green onions, basil, salt, and pepper and sauté until vegetables are tender, about 4 minutes.

3. Beat together eggs and milk and pour over vegetables in skillet over medium-high heat.

4. Arrange chunks of salmon over top of egg-vegetable mixture in the skillet.

5. Reduce to medium-low heat, cover, and cook until eggs are set, about 15 minutes.

RATATOUILLE WITH SCRAMBLED EGGS

Serves 6 to 8

2	cloves garlic, crushed and minced
1	onion, diced
2	tablespoons cold-pressed, extra-virgin olive oil or organic canola oil
2	zucchini, sliced
1	green bell pepper, diced
1	Japanese/Chinese eggplant, sliced
2	tomatoes, diced
1	teaspoon salt
2	tablespoons finely chopped fresh flat-leaf parsley leaves
2	teaspoons dried basil
1	teaspoon dried oregano
4	tablespoons cold-pressed, extra-virgin olive oil or organic canola oil
1	teaspoon salt
1	500-gram carton Egg Creations Original (liquid egg white)

1. In a skillet, sauté garlic and onion in olive oil or canola oil for 1–2 minutes over medium heat.

2. Add zucchini and bell pepper and continue to sauté over medium heat for another 3–4 minutes.

3. Add eggplant and continue to sauté over medium heat for another 5 minutes until all the vegetables are tender.

4. Add tomatoes, salt, and all the herbs. Mix into vegetable mixture well and set aside.

5. In a skillet, heat 2 tablespoons olive oil or canola oil over medium heat. Pour in half the carton of Egg Creations Original liquid egg white and 1/2 teaspoon of salt. As the mixture begins to cook, gently move spatula across the skillet to form large, soft curds. Cook until eggs are set but still moist. Set aside. Repeat to finish cooking rest of eggs.

6. Place scrambled eggs on a large plate and top with ratatouille.

RED PEPPER AND MUSHROOM STUFFED OMELET

SERVES 1

1	clove garlic, crushed and minced
1/2	onion, diced
1	tablespoon cold-pressed, extra-virgin olive oil or organic canola oil
1/2	cup thinly sliced cremini (brown) mushrooms
1/2	sweet red pepper, very finely diced
1/2	teaspoon salt
2	omega-3 eggs
2	tablespoons vanilla rice milk (e.g., Rice Dream)
1/2	teaspoon salt
	Pinch pepper
1/4	cup finely chopped fresh flat-leaf parsley leaves
1	tablespoon cold-pressed, extra-virgin olive oil or organic canola oil

1. In a skillet, sauté garlic and half the diced onions in 1 tablespoon olive oil or canola oil for 1–2 minutes over medium heat.

2. Add mushrooms, half the diced sweet red pepper, and 1/2 teaspoon salt, and sauté until vegetables are tender, about 3 minutes. Remove the mixture from the pan. Cover and keep warm.

3. In a small bowl, beat together eggs, milk, salt and pepper. Add the parsley leaves, remaining onions, and remaining diced sweet peppers to the egg mixture.

4. Heat 1 tablespoon olive oil or canola oil in a skillet over medium-high heat and pour the egg mixture into the skillet. Reduce heat to medium-low, cover, and cook until eggs are set, about 4 minutes.

5. When eggs are cooked through, top with reserved mushroom-red-pepper mixture on one half of the omelet. Fold omelet in half and slide from skillet onto plate.

About the Ingredients

Balsamic vinegar: This is a dark vinegar made from white trebbiano
grapes with an intense, rich flavor that is both sweet and salty,
sharp, and acidic.

Barley: This is a cereal grain that has a nutty flavor and chewy,
pasta-like consistency. It is a great addition to soups, stews,
and salads since it really soaks up the flavors used in the broth
or dressing. It is rich in selenium and is an excellent source of
soluble fiber, which makes it a low-glycemic-index food—in fact,
barley has one of the lowest glycemic-index values of any food.
It is also especially rich in beta-glucans, which helps to lower
cholesterol. Cup for cup, it provides almost double the amount
of fiber as brown rice. Choose pot barley and not pearled barley—the pearled form has been milled so that its fiber-rich bran
layer has been removed. Pot barley is not as intensely milled and
therefore retains some of its bran.

Basil: This highly fragrant herb has a minty, sweet flavor with citrus
overtones and is most aromatic when used fresh. The fresh herb
should be added at the last minute of cooking as prolonged heat
destroys the flavor very quickly.

Bay leaf: This herb has a deep and savory aroma that helps to add
depth and flavor to foods and enhances the taste of any soup,
stew, or sauce it is added to.

Brown rice: Since it retains the outer bran layer containing most
of the grain's fiber, vitamins, and minerals, brown rice is far
more nutritious than white rice. It has a mildly nutty flavor and
is chewier than white rice. For those who don't like the taste of
brown rice but want the nutritional benefits, try substituting half
the white rice in a recipe for brown rice with a more gradual
palate change.

Burdock root (gobo): This herb is commonly used in both Western
and Asian medicines to treat skin problems, such as acne,
eczema, or psoriasis. It supports the liver, cleanses the blood,
and enhances elimination through the bile and bowels. It can
be enjoyed as a food as it is available in the vegetable section of

most Asian markets. Burdock root has a strong, sweet, earthy taste and can be prepared and eaten almost exactly like carrots.

Butternut squash: This large pear-shaped vegetable with golden-yellow skin takes a bit of time to chop and peel. However, the orange flesh when cooked has a delectable rich, sweet, creamy flavor that is worth the effort. It is also rich in beta-carotene, vitamin C, and fiber. Many grocery stores also sell precut butternut squash cubes.

Cherry tomatoes: These are smaller than the garden variety of tomato and are sweeter, making them an excellent choice used raw in salads.

Cilantro: Also known as **coriander** or **Chinese parlsey**. This herb looks similar to flat-leaf parsley but tastes very different. It gives a wonderful, tangy, citrus flavor to recipes and can be used liberally when you want to add some zest to a dish. Always add it toward the end of cooking or just before serving since the flavor decreases with cooking.

Cremini mushrooms: Also known as **Italian mushrooms** or **brown mushrooms**. Mushrooms add a wonderful rich, earthy flavor to many dishes. They are also a source of vitamins B1, B2, and B3. Cremini mushrooms are closely related to common white mushrooms, but are richer in flavor. **Portobello mushrooms** are simply large cremini mushrooms. You may substitute any mushrooms in the recipes below, depending on your tastes.

Cumin: This spice has a distinctive strong, warm, and musty flavor. It is often found in Indian and Mexican cuisines and is a key ingredient in curry and chili powders.

Dill: Also known as dill weed, the wispy feathery leaves of this herb give a light, delicate and aromatic flavor to a dish.

Edamame: Also known as **green soybeans**, they are readily available frozen, both in the pod and shelled, in Asian food stores and more recently in many health food stores and regular grocery stores. They are young, immature soybeans that cook very quickly—simply boil in lightly salted water for five to ten minutes until tender. They can be eaten on their own as a side dish or added to other recipes.

Ginger root: Its spicy, sweet aroma and flavor have made it a favorite in cuisines around the world. But it is not just a culinary plant, it also has many medicinal properties—it has been shown to lower cholesterol, prevent blood clots by decreasing platelet aggregation, and has potent anti-inflammatory and antinausea properties.

Kale: This is one of the most highly nutritious vegetables, rich in vitamins, antioxidants, fiber, and calcium. It's no wonder since it belongs to the *Brassica* family, the same family that nutrient powerhouse vegetables such as broccoli, cabbage, and Brussels sprouts belong to. The leaves and stalk are both edible and are delicious simply sautéed with garlic and olive oil. Many recipes call for leaves only since the stalk can be fibrous and hard if not cooked long enough or with older kale plants.

Leek: Belonging to the same family as onions and garlic (*Allium*), leeks contain many of the same health-promoting compounds found to be beneficial for cholesterol, blood pressure, and blood thinning. They have a more delicate and sweet taste than onions and garlic and add a more subtle flavor to recipes without overpowering them.

Mackerel: This fish is very high in omega-3s and is best prepared fresh—straight from store to pan. Fresh mackerel is very perishable, so if you are not eating it that day, you must store it on ice in the coldest part of the refrigerator and cover it with foil or plastic wrap and prepare it within two days. Otherwise, it will quickly develop a fishy flavor and go rancid. Don't purchase king mackerel, as it is one of the fish that is highest in mercury. The secret to cooking mackerel is not to overcook. It will be cooked when its flesh becomes opaque but still moist and can easily be pierced by a fork.

Millet: This grain is one of the main ingredients in birdseed. However, it is also a food staple in Asia, Africa, and India. The taste of this gluten-free grain can vary significantly depending on the amount of water used during cooking. For a softer and creamier consistency, add more water. For a drier and fluffier consistency, add less. You can also bring out its subtle nutty flavor by lightly roasting the grain in a dry pan before cooking.

Miso: This salty paste is a traditional Japanese food made by fermenting soybeans with salt and other grains, such as rice, wheat, or barley. It is a source of B vitamins, isoflavones, and enzymes. There are many varieties, but, in general, the darker the color, the saltier the taste; and the lighter the color, the sweeter and less salty the taste. Use it sparingly—a little miso will add a salty taste to any dish it is added to.

Okra: Not everyone enjoys the texture of okra. However, its unique texture is what contributes to its health benefits. When cut and cooked, okra releases a gummy substance, known as mucilage, and round edible seeds. This mucilage acts as a thickening agent in soups, stews, and gumbos and is also a source of soluble fiber which is known to lower cholesterol and blood glucose.

Oregano: This is an herb with a bold, peppery taste, but in small amounts it can add a warm, balsamic flavor to a dish. The dried herb is more flavorful than the fresh.

Oyster mushrooms: Now cultivated and widely available, the oyster mushroom is easy to spot with its graceful, shell-shaped cap. It has a delicate, mild flavor suitable for those who desire less of the "earthy" taste that mushrooms can impart to a dish.

Paprika: This spice is made from dried, ground sweet red peppers and adds a sweet and mildly spicy flavor to dishes, as well as an attractive color.

Parsley: The two most common varieties are the flat-leafed Italian parsley and the bushy curly parsley. Both have a fresh and subtle celery taste. However, the Italian variety has a richer, more fragrant taste that stands up better when used in cooking versus the curly variety, which is preferred for garnishes or used raw in salads.

Portobello mushrooms: See **cremini mushrooms** above.

Quinoa: This light, fluffy grain with a slightly nutty flavor is native to the Andes mountains in South America. It is a favorite of vegetarians as it is one of the few vegetable sources of complete protein, containing a balance of all the essential amino acids. It is also a gluten-free grain, easy to digest, and quick to cook.

Rice vinegar: This is a milder and sweeter alternative to regular vinegar. It is good in sweet-and-sour dishes, for pickling vegetables, and generally works well in stir-fries.

Rosemary: This herb has leaves that look like pine needles and has a strong pine-like flavor. Be judicious when using rosemary in recipes because its flavor can dominate a dish and cause it to become bitter when used in excess.

Salmon: Salmon is among the fish highest in omega-3s. Choose wild Pacific salmon when possible as opposed to farmed Atlantic salmon—they are fed fishmeal, which studies show is contaminated with PCBs, dioxins, and organochlorines. Furthermore, farmed salmon is much higher in the omega-6 fatty acids we are overconsuming.

Sherry: Regular sherry can replace cooking sherry in any recipe. It will subtly enhance the flavor of any dish, especially stir-fries and rice, and can also be used as a marinade.

Shiitake mushrooms: Shiitake mushrooms have a rich, smokey flavor and can be found fresh or dried. They are more commonly found dried as the dried form helps to bring out their flavor. Dried mushrooms must be rehydrated by soaking them in water before cooking. The stems of shiitake are rarely used because they are harder and take longer to cook than the soft fleshy caps. They have been used medicinally in China for more than six thousand years and are widely studied today due to their documented immune-supporting health benefits.

Sweet Potatoes: Although white potatoes have a high glycemic index/load, sweet potatoes are a low-glycemic-index food, so enjoy them as a healthy source of complex carbohydrates. They are rich in beta-carotene (the precursor to vitamin A), containing twice the daily requirement of this vitamin and are a great source of fiber. Try replacing them in any favorite recipe that calls for white potatoes to reap added health benefits.

Swiss Chard: This is a superb vegetable rich in vitamins and minerals. Both the dark green leaves and stalk (which vary from white, yellow, or red) are edible and taste like a cross between beets and spinach. Use it in any recipe that calls for spinach, but cook it a little longer.

Tempeh: Like tofu, tempeh is made from soy, but because it is made from the whole soybean, it has a much higher protein content and gives a stronger flavor and texture to recipes. Tempeh is made from a controlled fermented process that binds whole cooked soybeans into block-like cakes. It has a firm texture and nutty, mushroom flavor and can be marinated, puréed, grilled, steamed, or fried, as well as sliced, diced, or crumbled.

Thyme: This herb has a strong, robust flavor with hints of pine. Use it sparingly, as it can overwhelm other flavors in the dish if used too liberally.

Tofu: Also known as bean curd, tofu is made by curdling soy milk with a coagulant. It is found labeled as silken, soft, medium, firm, or extra-firm, depending on how much liquid has been extracted. The firmer the tofu, the more protein it contains, but the more dense in consistency. Choose silken, soft, or medium-firm tofu and marinate it before adding to recipes to boost the flavor—this will help those whose palates are not accustomed to the flavor and texture of tofu.

Tomato paste: This thick paste is made from ripened tomatoes whose skin and seeds have been removed. It is often used as a base for pizza sauce but can also be used to infuse a tomato flavor into other dishes without the extra liquid common with using tomato sauce or fresh tomatoes.

Turmeric: This spice will cause your dish to turn golden yellow in color and will give it a distinct warm and mustardy taste. It is a key ingredient in curry powder and has potent anti-inflammatory and anticancer properties.

Sun-dried tomatoes: These are halved or quartered fresh tomatoes that have been left to dry in the sun to intensify their flavor. They have a strong smoky flavor and a pleasant, chewy texture. Those marinated in oil can be used directly, while those that are not must be rehydrated before using.

White wine vinegar: This light, flavorful, and fruity vinegar combines well with salads, sauces, and dressings.

Wild rice: Despite its name, this woodsy-flavored, slightly chewy grain is not actually related to rice. Instead, it is the seed of an

aquatic grass that grows in shallow water in marshes and along
the shores of rivers and streams. It has fewer calories and 50 percent more protein than white rice and is a good source of fiber.
It tends to be more expensive than other types of rice because of
the labor-intensive hand harvesting. But its excellent nutritional
profile and natural growth without chemicals or additives make it
a grain worth trying.

Afterword: In Appreciation of Dr. John H. Stokes

There is a dusty old textbook sitting in the University of Chicago library; thousands of students have walked past it over the years without paying it any mind. In fact, until Dr. Logan signed the book out as an interlibrary loan in September 2006, there was no record of its being signed out since February 15, 1960. The book is called *Fundamentals of Medical Dermatology* (University of Pennsylvania, Department of Dermatology Book Fund, 1942), by legendary dermatologist Dr. John H. Stokes. One might think an old book like that would offer very little to modern dermatology practice, especially with its newly patented skin creams and futuristic laser technology. Yet when we worked our way through the book, we were stunned by the content and realized quickly that John Stokes was a genius. *Fundamentals of Medical Dermatology* is, in many ways, as valuable today as it was the year it was published.

Born in Germany in 1885, John Stokes earned his undergraduate and medical degrees at the University of Michigan. He also trained in dermatology at the University of Michigan and went on to help open the dermatology section of the famous Mayo Clinic. He was convinced of a relationship between the psyche and skin conditions, so it was no surprise that he would make history as the first physician to employ the use of social workers in any Mayo Clinic department. In 1924 he left the Mayo Clinic to take charge of the University of Pennsylvania dermatology section. In addition to his teaching and

administrative responsibilities, Dr. Stokes took on a large and successful clinical dermatology practice. Patients would travel great distances
to meet with this highly regarded dermatologist.

His practice was described by colleague Dr. Herman Beerman
(writing in the *Journal of the American Academy of Dermatology*, 1983):
"He handled his patients in a holistic manner long before this phi-
losophy of medicine, and especially cutaneous [skin] medicine, was
in vogue." Detailed history-taking was extremely important in assessments, including the lifestyle of the individual. His psychotherapeutic
approach was unrivaled, and dietary influences on skin conditions,
including acne, were taken seriously. The normal function of the gastrointestinal tract and the bacterial microflora residing in the gut were
also important considerations for Dr. Stokes.

John Hinchman Stokes passed away on February 23, 1961, yet his
teachings live on, albeit in the few remaining dusty textbooks that sit
in the holdings of some fortunate science libraries. Known by students
as "The Blue Book" due to its deep blue color, *Fundamentals of Medical
Dermatology* remains a superb and relevant piece of dermatologic history. Here's why:

1. The influence of the gastrointestinal system on skin conditions
   is described on pages 206–11, including the value of correcting
   intestinal stasis (constipation) and the use of fiber-rich foods
   as well as probiotics (acidophilus). We now know, some sixty-
   plus years later, that constipation does influence inflammatory
   markers beyond the gut, and probiotics, including various
   strains of *Lactobacillus*, have been documented in well-designed
   clinical trials to be of value in skin conditions. Dr. Stokes also
   makes note of the major influence of nervous stress on the gastrointestinal tract—referring to the GI tract as "an emotional
   highway" long before the volumes of research would prove it
   to be so.

2. The influence of a low-carbohydrate diet on skin conditions is
   described on pages 211–13. Long before the Zone and South
   Beach Diets, Dr. Stokes was advocating a reduction in the overconsumption of simple carbohydrates without the valuable fiber.
   He makes note of the vastly greater consumption of simple carbohydrates (including fountain drinks, candy and candy bars, ice

cream, etc.) in North America compared to other regions. He makes the distinction, long before *whole grains* and *dietary fiber* were buzzwords, that the carbohydrates in vegetables are broken down differently (compared to sweets) due to the presence of the fiber. On page 213, he states, "Substitute whole wheat or graham bread or rolls, for white flour products." Decades before the USDA's 1991 establishment of the five-a-day campaign for three servings of vegetables and two servings of fruit daily, Dr. Stokes advised patients to "eat at least three vegetables and a salad a day." Clearly, he had no clue in 1942 that vegetables are loaded with antioxidant phytochemicals, many of which are now known to work efficiently in the human skin. He also had no idea of how fiber-rich whole grains and fruits and vegetables can influence inflammation and even androgen levels. Amazingly, there was also the recommendation that pastries, puddings, fruit juices, and other sweet snacks should be substituted with "whole fruits." Not only are whole fruits loaded with colorful phytochemicals, they also contain fiber to prevent blood-sugar spiking. Obviously, when Dr. Stokes penned *Fundamentals of Medical Dermatology*, he had no idea of the physiological consequences of insulin and insulin-like growth hormone stimulation at the sebaceous gland!

3. An entire section, pages 219–26, is devoted to the importance of the psyche and psychotherapeutic interventions in dermatology. Assessment of the stressors and emotional background was vital to patient care as taught by Dr. Stokes. The section is a template for modern mind-body medicine. He gives advice on what is now termed "progressive muscular relaxation"; he discusses giving up the use of *must* in the vocabulary, a word that often gets us into trouble with workload, demands, and overall stress. He focused on recognition of the signs of tension, and before mindfulness meditation was a well-defined modality within mind-body medicine, he underscored the importance of "living in the moment." He suggests therapeutic walking while thinking only of the present and avoiding past ruminations and future fears. He recommends conscious awareness of the trees, clouds, and other natural sights when walking. This is exactly what mindfulness

meditation is all about, and these concepts remain central to mind-body medicine and its influence on human health. Long before yoga studios became a part of every suburban strip mall, John Stokes was describing the benefit of gentle exercise in dermatology. He was leery of competition exercises and overtraining, which he felt were not as effective in lowering stress as activities such as walking—this was long before the research on increased androgens and oxidative stress in competition and overtraining (versus more passive exercise). He recognized the importance of sleep for healthy skin, and even though drugs for sleep were around at the time, he felt they should be used only as a last resort—not before environmental-emotional aspects were addressed first. About forty years before Dr. Judith Wurtman showed that a small amount of carbohydrate (taken away from protein-rich foods) can boost tryptophan and serotonin levels, Dr. Stokes advocated for a small amount of carbohydrate to help induce sleep. He also recommended the now well-known advice to get up and perform some activities when one cannot sleep—and the stress-reducing techniques were emphasized to help remove the influence of worry/anxiety on sleep. We now know that lack of quality sleep is reported to be one of the worst offenders when it comes to acne flare-ups. Over half of patients state that lack of sleep makes acne worse—not surprising, since stress, lack of sleep, and poor dietary choices often go hand in hand.

4. So those were the general rules for healthy skin for all—then there is the specific section on acne. Here Dr. Stokes once again discusses the importance of sleep, intestinal microflora (i.e., making sure we have enough of the good bacteria), nutrition, overconsumption of simple carbohydrates and fats, stress, and the mental state of the patient. With the recently published works on acne and all of these topics, we find it incredible that he was on the right track with so many diet-lifestyle factors. We were particularly struck by one line on page 398, where he suggests that clinicians should be on the lookout for "broken hearts" in cases of acne—some fifty years before Dr. C. I. Harrington from the

Royal Hallamshire Hospital in the United Kingdom reported on cases of adult acne in women after experiencing the breakup of their marriages.

In the two decades following the publication of *Fundamentals of Medical Dermatology*, there occurred the dawning of a new era in dermatology. During this time there was a major transition of dermatological thinking: from an art to a science. There is certainly nothing wrong with the pursuit of progressive science; yet, in the process, the documented lifestyle factors were tossed out like a moldy loaf of bread. Dermatology set out, with good reason, to establish itself as a sophisticated science—diet and intangible psychosocial issues were not part of that process. Diet became the stuff of high school home economics class, far removed from "real" scientific affairs. Some already viewed dermatologists, as Jerry Seinfeld would playfully put it, as "one step up from the Clinique counter." Diet, carrying on about two salads and a vegetable, this business of living in the moment, and the vagaries of lifestyle counseling? Come on now, in a profession striving for respect, this was not going to impress the neurosurgeon at the cocktail party. The explosion in science would certainly make dermatology a cutting-edge, scientific profession. However, advances in nutritional medicine would also uncover detailed physiological pathways of dietary influences in acne. Mind-body medicine, as it would come to be called, also showed terrific scientific advances that would justify its inclusion in virtually all chronic illnesses.

While the lifestyle factors that Dr. Stokes advocated in the 1940s were not scientifically assessed until recent years, he was not unscientific; it was he, after all, and a select group of colleagues who established the Society for Investigative Dermatology. This group, established in 1937, was charged with the detailed scientific exploration of the skin and its anatomy and physiology. The investigations of this group have led to the development of effective medications and other treatments, as well as a much greater understanding of the intricate barrier that separates us from the outside world.

In the last several years, the research on psychological stress and acne has been published, the research on glycemic foods and acne was published, and the Harvard studies on diet (milk) and others on anger/emotions and acne have followed. So, too, has research on oxidative stress and inflammation shed light on potential nutritional pathways of influence on acne. As the research on lifestyle factors in skin diseases, and acne in particular, starts to finally gain momentum, many of the teachings of Dr. Stokes are being validated.

In October 2005, an entire issue of the prestigious journal *Dermatologic Clinics* was devoted to psychosocial factors in skin diseases. As Dr. M. A. Gupta stated in the editorial preface of the journal, psychosocial factors in skin disorders "constitute an important component of treatment outcome." That is exactly what Dr. Stokes was saying in 1942, and that is obviously what he was thinking in November 1921 when he called for a social worker to be present in the Mayo Clinic dermatology section. *Fundamentals of Medical Dermatology* is heading toward its seventieth birthday, but it remains a classic and should never be forgotten; it is the foundation and inspiration for what we now know about the modern clear skin diet. Our version of *The Clear Skin Diet* was in many ways already written in 1942, we have simply filled in the scientific blanks Dr. Stokes did not have the clues for some sixty-five years ago.

John H. Stokes M.D.—a genius who helped to build modern dermatology.

References

Abdou et al. 2006. Relaxation and immunity enhancement effects of gamma-amino-butyric acid (GABA) administration in humans. *Biofactors* 26 (3): 201–8.

Acharya. 1990. Vitamin E (tocoferol acetate) in the treatment of adolescent acne. *J Assoc Physicians India* 38 (2): 189–90.

Adachi et al. 2006. Epigallocatechin gallate attenuates acute stress responses through GABAergic system in the brain. *Eur J Pharmacol* 531 (1–3): 171–75.

Adams et al. 1985. Long-term antibiotic therapy for acne vulgaris: Effects on the bowel flora of patients and their relatives. *J Invest Dermatol* 85 (1): 35–37.

Adams et al. 2006. Status of nutrition education in medical schools. *Am J Clin Nutr* 83 (4): 941S–944S.

Adebamowo et al. 2005. High school dietary dairy intake and teenage acne. *J Am Acad Dermatol* 52 (2): 207–14.

Adebamowo et al. 2006. Milk consumption and acne in adolescent girls. *Dermatol Online J* 12 (4): 1.

Aikawa et al. 1956. The effects of glucuronic acid on acne vulgaris. *Tohoku J Exp Med* 64 (3–4): 301–3.

Ajani et al. 2004. Dietary fiber and C-reactive protein: Findings from national health and nutrition examination survey data. *J Nutr* 134 (5): 1181–85.

Akhundov et al. 1993. Psychoregulating role of nicotinamide. *Biull Eksp Biol Med* 115 (5): 487–91.

Alestas et al. 2006. Enzymes involved in the biosynthesis of leukotriene B4 and prostaglandin E2 are active in sebaceous glands. *J Mol Med* 84 (1): 75–87.

Amado et al. 2006. The prevalence of acne in the north of Portugal. *J Eur Acad Dermatol Venereol* 20 (10): 1287–95.

Anderson. 1971. Foods as the cause of acne. *Am Fam Physician* 3 (3): 102–3.

Anderson. 2004. An update on the effects of playing violent video games. *J Adolesc* 27 (1): 113–22.

Anderson. 2005. A preliminary investigation of the enzymatic inhibition of 5alpha-reduction and growth of prostatic carcinoma cell line LNCap-FGC by natural astaxanthin and Saw Palmetto lipid extract in vitro. *J Herb Pharmacother* 5 (1): 17–26.

Andersen et al. 2006. Consumption of coffee is associated with reduced risk of death attributed to inflammatory and cardiovascular diseases in the Iowa Women's Health Study. *Am J Clin Nutr* 83 (5): 1039–46.

Andrew et al. 2005. The contribution of visceral adipose tissue to splanchnic cortisol production in healthy humans. *Diabetes* 54 (5): 1364–70.

Angel. 1996. Drug advertisements and prescribing. *Lancet* 348 (9039): 1452–53.

Angel. 2003. Industry sponsorship of continuing medical education. *JAMA* 290 (9): 1149–50.

Anonymous. 2004. Harvard Medical School. Coffee: for most, it's safe. Coffee has been blamed for everything from moral turpitude to cancer. But none of the bad raps have stuck. Coffee may even be good for you. *Harv Women's Health Watch* 12 (1): 2–4.

Arican et al. 2005. Oxidative stress in patients with acne vulgaris. *Mediators Inflamm* (6): 380–84.

Arranz et al. 2007. Impairment of several immune functions in anxious women. *J Psychosom* 62 (1): 1–8.

Atanasov et al. 2006. Coffee inhibits the reactivation of glucocorticoids by 11beta-hydroxysteroid dehydrogenase type 1: A glucocorticoid connection in the anti-diabetic action of coffee? *FEBS Lett* 580 (17): 4081–85.

August et al. 1999. Ingestion of green tea rapidly decreases prostaglandin E2 levels in rectal mucosa in humans. *Cancer Epidemiol Biomarkers Prev* 8 (8): 709–13.

Ayers and Mihan. 1978. Acne vulgaris and lipid peroxidation: New concepts in pathogenesis and treatment. *Int J Dermatol* 17 (4): 305–7.

Ayers and Mihan. 1981. Acne vulgaris: Therapy directed at pathophysiologic defects. *Cutis* 28 (1): 41–42.

Baharav et al. 2004. Lactobacillus GG bacteria ameliorate arthritis in Lewis rats. *J Nutr* 134 (8): 1964–69.

Baker. 1999. Cupric oxide should not be used as a copper supplement for either animals or humans. *J Nutr* 129 (12): 2278–79.

Bartlett. Clinical practice. 2002. Antibiotic-associated diarrhea. *N Engl J Med* 346 (5): 334–39.

Bayen et al. 2005. Effect of cooking on the loss of persistent organic pollutants from salmon. *J Toxicol Environ Health A* 68 (4): 253–65.

Beddoe and Murphy. 2004. Does mindfulness decrease stress and foster empathy among nursing students? *J Nurs Educ* 43 (7): 305–12.

Beerman. 1983. John Hinchman Stokes, M.D.: An appreciation. *J Am Acad Dermatol* 9 (2): 321–34.

Bellisle et al. 2004. Non food-related environmental stimuli induce increased meal intake in healthy women: Comparison of television viewing versus listening to a recorded story in laboratory settings. *Appetite* 3 (2): 175–80.

Bendiner E. 1974. Disastrous trade-off: Eskimo health for white civilization. *Hosp Pract* 9:156–89.

Benno et al. 1986. Comparison of the fecal microflora in rural Japanese and urban Canadians. *Microbiol Immunol* 30 (6): 521–32.

Benno et al. 1989. Comparison of fecal microflora of elderly persons in rural and urban areas of Japan. *Appl Environ Microbiol* 55 (5): 1100–1105.

Benson. 2005. Are you working too hard? A conversation with mind/body researcher Herbert Benson. *Harv Bus Rev* 83 (11): 53–58, 165.

Benton. 2002. Selenium intake, mood and other aspects of psychological functioning. *Nutr Neurosci* 5 (6): 363–74.

Benton et al. 2006. Impact of consuming a milk drink containing a probiotic on mood and cognition. *Eur J Clin Nut* (December) [Epub ahead of print].

Berrino et al. 2001. Reducing bioavailable sex hormones through a comprehensive change in diet: The diet and androgens (DIANA) randomized trial. *Cancer Epidemiol Biomarkers Prev* 10 (1): 25–33.

Biro et al. 2003. Clinical implications of thermal therapy in lifestyle-related diseases. *Exp Biol Med* (Maywood) 228 (10): 1245–49.

Blomhoff et al. 2006. Health benefits of nuts: Potential role of antioxidants. *Br J Nutr* 96 (November; Suppl 2): S52–60.

Bourne and Jacobs. 1956. Observations on acne, seborrhoea, and obesity. *Br Med J* 1 (4978): 1268–70.

Bowe, et al. 2007. Body dysmorphic disorder symptons among patients with acne vulgaris. *J Am Acad Dermatol* (May 9) [Epub ahead of print].

Bradbury et al. 2004. An adaptogenic role for omega-3 fatty acids in stress; a randomized placebo controlled double blind intervention study (pilot) [ISRCTN22569553]. *Nutr J* 3 (November): 20.

Bradbury et al. 2004. Are low-fat diets associated with stress? *Int J Nat Med* 1:33–42.

Bremner et al. 2005. Functional brain imaging alterations in acne patients treated with isotretinoin. *Am J Psychiatry* 162 (5): 983–91.

Brown and Ryan. 2003. The benefits of being present: Mindfulness and its role in psychological well-being. *J Pers Soc Psychol* 84 (4): 822–48.

Bulbena et al. 2005. Panic anxiety, under the weather? *Int J Biometeorol* 49 (4): 238–43.

Burger et al. 2003. Effect of deep-frying fish on risk from mercury. *J Toxicol Environ Health A* 66 (9): 817–28.

Buydens et al. 2005. N-3 polyunsaturated fatty acids decrease feelings of anger in a population of substance abusers. *Neuropsychopharmacology* 30 (1): S87–S88.

Calder. 2006. N-3 polyunsaturated fatty acids, inflammation, and inflammatory diseases. *Am J Clin Nutr* 83 (6 Suppl): 1505S–1519S.

Callaghan. 2004. Exercise: A neglected intervention in mental health care? *J Psychiatr Mental Health Nurs* 11:476–83.

Campbell et al. 2006. Serum testosterone is reduced following short-term phytofluene, lycopene, or tomato powder consumption in F344 rats. *J Nutr* 136 (11): 2813–19.

Campione et al. 2006. Severe acne successfully treated with etanercept. *Acta Derm Venereol* 86 (3): 256–57.

Cappel et al. 2005. Correlation between serum levels of insulin-like growth factor 1, dehydroepiandrosterone sulfate, and dihydrotestosterone and acne lesion counts in adult women. *Arch Derm* 141:333–38.

Card et al. 2004. Antibiotic use and the development of Crohn's disease. *Gut* 53 (2): 246–50.

Caris-Veyrat et al. 2004. Influence of organic versus conventional agricultural practice on the antioxidant microconstituent content of tomatoes and derived purees; consequences on antioxidant plasma status in humans. *J Agric Food Chem* 52 (21): 6503–9.

Cartwright et al. 2003. Stress and dietary practices in adolescents. *Health Psychol* 22 (4): 362–69.

Cernerud and Olsson. 2004. Humor seen from a public health perspective. *Scan J Public Health* 32:396–98.

Chesley. 2005. Blurring boundaries? Linking technology use, spillover, individual distress, and family satisfaction. *J Marriage Fam* 67:1237–48.

Chiu et al. 2003. The response of skin disease to stress: Changes in the severity of acne vulgaris as affected by examination stress. *Arch Dermatol* 139 (7): 897–900.

Choi et al. 2006. A single-blinded, randomized, controlled clinical trial evaluating the effect of face washing on acne vulgaris. *Pediatr Dermatol* 23 (5): 421–27.

Coeuret et al. 2004. Numbers and strains of lactobacilli in some probiotic products. *Int J Food Microbiol* 97 (2): 147–56.

Cohen and Cohen. 1958. Pustular acne, staphyloderma and its treatment with tolbutamide. *Can Med Assoc J* 80 (8): 629–32.

Cohen et al. 1993. Mechanisms of chromium carcinogenicity and toxicity. *Crit Rev Toxicol* 23 (3): 255–81.

1999. Comparison of n-3 polyunsaturated fatty acids from vegetable oils, meat, and fish in raising platelet eicosapentaenoic acid levels in humans. *Lipids* (34 Suppl): S309.

Cordain et al. 2002. Acne vulgaris: A disease of Western civilization. *Arch Dermatol* 138 (12): 1584–90.

Cordain et al. 2005. Origins and evolution of the Western diet: Health implications for the 21st century. *Am J Clin Nutr* 81 (2): 341–54.

Craig and Beck. 1999. Phytochemicals: Health Protective Effects. *Can J Diet Pract Res* 60 (2): 78–84.

Cruickshank et al. 1963. Subclinical glycosuria in acne vulgaris. *Br J Dermatol* 75 (August–September): 363–66.

Danby. 2007. Acne and iodine: Reply. *J Am Acad Dermatol* 56 (1): 164–65.

Danby FW. 2003. Night blindness, vitamin A deficiency, and isotretinoin psycho-toxicity. *Dermatology Online Journal* 9 (5): 30

Daughton. 2002. Environmental stewardship and drugs as pollutants. *Lancet* 360 (9339): 1035–36.

Davidson et al. 2003. Alterations in brain and immune function produced by mindfulness meditation. *Psychosom Med* 65 (4): 564–70.

Denomme et al. 2005. Directly quantitated dietary (n-3) fatty acid intakes of pregnant Canadian women are lower than current dietary recommendations. *J Nutr* 135 (2): 206–11.

Deuschle et al. 1997. Insulin-like growth factor-I (IGF-I) plasma concentrations are increased in depressed patients. *Psychoneuroendocrinology* 22 (7): 493–503.

Docherty et al. 2005. A double-blind, placebo-controlled, exploratory trial of chromium picolinate in atypical depression: Effect on carbohydrate craving. *J Psychiatr Pract* 11 (5): 302–14.

Dolara et al. 2005. Red wine polyphenols influence carcinogenesis, intestinal microflora, oxidative damage and gene expression profiles of colonic mucosa in F344 rats. *Mutat Res* 591 (1–2): 237–46.

Dreno et al. 1989. Low doses of zinc gluconate for inflammatory acne. *Acta Derm Venereo* 69 (6): 541–43.

Dreno et al. 2005. Effect of zinc gluconate on propionibacterium acnes resistance to erythromycin in patients with inflammatory acne: In vitro and in vivo study. *Eur J Dermatol* 15 (3): 152–55.

Ebner et al. 2006. The role of substance P in stress and anxiety responses. *Amino Acids* 31 (3): 251–72.

Ekanayake-Mudiyanselage et al. 2004. Oral supplementation with all-Rac- and RRR-alpha-tocopherol increases vitamin E levels in human sebum after a latency period of 14-21 days. *Ann N Y Acad Sci* 1031 (December): 184–94.

El-Akawi et al. 2006. Does the plasma level of vitamins A and E affect acne condition? *Clin Exp Dermatol* 31 (3): 430–34.

Elkin and Rosch. 1990. Promoting mental health at the workplace. *Occup Med* 5:739–54.

Eller et al. 2006. Psychosocial factors at home and at work and levels of salivary cortisol. *Biol Psychol* 73 (3): 280–87.

Esposito and Giugliano. 2006. Whole-grain intake cools down inflammation. *Am J Clin Nutr* 83 (6): 1440–41.

Evans et al. 2005. Teenage acne is influenced by genetic factors. *Br J Dermatol* 152 (3): 579–81.

Fakhrzadeh et al. 2005. The effects of consumption of omega3 fatty acid-enriched eggs on insulin and CRP. *Nutr Metab Cardiovasc Dis* 15 (4): 329–30.

Fallon and Enig. 2000. *Nourishing Traditions*, 2nd ed. Washington, DC: New Trends Publishing.

Farrar and Ingham. 2004. Acne: Inflammation. *Clin Dermatol* 22 (5): 380–84.

Feldman et al. 2004. Diagnosis and treatment of acne. *Am Fam Physician* 69 (9): 2123–30.

Field et al. 2002. Fibromyalgia pain and substance P decrease and sleep improves after massage therapy. *J Clin Rheumatol* 8 (2): 72–76.

Flynn et al. 2003. Inadequate physician knowledge of the effects of diet on blood lipids and lipoproteins. *Nutr J* 2 (December): 19.

Fontani et al. 2005. Cognitive and physiological effects of Omega-3 polyunsaturated fatty acid supplementation in healthy subjects. *Eur J Clin Invest* 5 (11): 691–99.

Fors et al. 2002. The effect of guided imagery and amitriptyline on daily fibromyalgia pain: A prospective, randomized, controlled trial. *J Psychiatr Res* 36 (3): 179–87.

Fox. 1999. The influence of physical activity on mental well-being. *Public Health Nutr* 2 (3A): 411–18.

Francis et al. 1988. Insulin-like growth factors 1 and 2 in bovine colostrum. Sequences and biological activities compared with those of a potent truncated form. *Biochem J* 251 (1): 95–103.

Fulton et al. 1969. Effect of chocolate on acne vulgaris. *JAMA* 210 (11): 2071–74.

Furukawa et al. 2004. Increased oxidative stress in obesity and its impact on metabolic syndrome. *J Clin Invest* 114 (12): 1752–61.

Galobardes et al. 2005. Has acne increased? Prevalence of acne history among university students between 1948 and 1968. The Glasgow Alumni Cohort Study. *Br J Dermatol* 152 (4): 824–25.

Galobardes et al. 2005. Acne in adolescence and cause-specific mortality: Lower coronary heart disease but higher prostate cancer mortality: The Glasgow Alumni Cohort Study. *Am J Epidemiol* 161 (12): 1094–1101.

Galvin et al. 2006. The relaxation response: Reducing stress and improving cognition in healthy aging adults. *Complement Ther Clin Pract* 12 (3): 186–91.

Gardner-Thorpe et al. 2003. Dietary supplements of soya flour lower serum testosterone concentrations and improve markers of oxidative stress in men. *Eur J Clin Nutr* 57 (1): 100–106.

Garner et al. 2003. Minocycline for acne vulgaris: Efficacy and safety. *Cochrane Database Syst Rev* (1): CD002086.

Gehring. 2004. Nicotinic acid/niacinamide and the skin. *J Cosmet Dermatol* 3 (2): 88–93.

Giltay et al. 2004. Docosahexaenoic acid concentrations are higher in women than in men because of estrogenic effects. *Am J Clin Nutr* 80 (5): 1167–74.

Gluck et al. 2003. Ingested probiotics reduce nasal colonization with pathogenic bacteria (Staphylococcus aureus, Streptococcus pneumoniae, and beta-hemolytic streptococci). *Am J Clin Nutr* 77 (2): 517–20.

Goel et al. 2005. Controlled trial of bright light and negative air ions for chronic depression. *Psychol Med* 35 (7): 945–55.

Goldberg et al. 2004. Advanced glycoxidation end products in commonly consumed foods. *J Am Diet Assoc* 104 (8): 1287–91.

Goldin et al. 1994. The effect of dietary fat and fiber on serum estrogen concentrations in premenopausal women under controlled dietary conditions. *Cancer* 74 (3 Suppl): 1125–31.

Golf et al. 1998. On the significance of magnesium in extreme physical stress. *Cardiovasc Drugs Ther* 12 (Suppl 2): 197–202.

Goolamali et al. 1974. Sebum excretion and melanocyte-stimulating hormone in hypoadrenalism. *J Invest Dermatol* 63 (3): 253–55.

Gordon and Porter. 2001. Minocycline induced lupus: Case series in the West of Scotland. *J Rheumatol* 28 (5): 1004–6.

Gore et al. 2003. Television viewing and snacking. *Eat Behav* 4 (4): 399–405.

Gortner et al. 2006. Benefits of expressive writing in lowering rumination and depressive symptoms. *Behav Ther* 37 (3): 292–303.

Grant and Anderson. 1965. Chocolate as a cause of acne: A dissenting view. *Mo Med* 62 (June): 459–60.

Grassi et al. 2005. Cocoa reduces blood pressure and insulin resistance and improves endothelium-dependent vasodilation in hypertensives. *Hypertension* 46 (2): 398–405.

Grebner et al. 2005. Working conditions and three types of well being: A longitudinal study with self-report and rating data. *J Occup Health Psychol* 10 (1): 31–43.

Green and Sinclair. 2001. Perceptions of acne vulgaris in final year medical student written examination answers. *Australas J Dermatol* 42 (2): 98–101.

Green et al. 2006. Red cell membrane omega-3 fatty acids are decreased in non-depressed patients with social anxiety disorder. *Eur Neuropsychopharmacol* 16 (2): 107–13.

Griesemer. 1978. Emotionally triggered disease in a dermatological practice. *Psychiatric Ann* 8 (8): 49–56.

Guenther et al. 2006. Most Americans eat much less than recommended amounts of fruits and vegetables. *J Am Diet Assoc* 106 (9): 1371–79.

Guillon et al. 1992. Minocycline-induced cell-mediated hypersensitivity pneumonitis. *Ann Intern Med* 117 (6): 476–81.

Gunnell et al. 2003. Are diet-prostate cancer associations mediated by the IGF axis? A cross-sectional analysis of diet, IGF-I and IGFBP-3 in healthy middle-aged men. *Br J Cancer* 88 (11): 1682–86.

Gupta. 2005. Preface: Psychocutaneous disease. *Dermatol Clin* 23: xiii–xiv.

Habito et al. 2000. Effects of replacing meat with soyabean in the diet on sex hormone concentrations in healthy adult males. *Br J Nutr* 84 (4): 557–63.

Haider and Shaw. 2004. Treatment of acne vulgaris. *JAMA* 292 (6): 726–35.

Halvorsen et al. 2006. Content of redox-active compounds (ie, antioxidants) in foods consumed in the United States. *Am J Clin Nutr* 84 (1): 95–135.

Hamalainen et al. 1984. Diet and serum sex hormones in healthy men. *J Steroid Biochem* 20 (1): 459–64.

Hamdaoui et al. 2005. Effect of green tea decoction on long-term iron, zinc and selenium status of rats. *Ann Nutr Metab* 49 (2): 118–24.

Hamilton, Terada, and Mestler. 1964. Greater tendency to acne in white American than in Japanese populations. *J Clin Endocrinol Metab* 24 (March): 267–72.

Hamilton-Miller et al. 1999. Public health issues arising from microbiological and labelling quality of foods and supplements containing probiotic microorganisms. *Public Health Nutr* 2 (2): 223–29.

Hara. 1997. Influence of tea catechins on the digestive tract. *J Cell Biochem Suppl* 27: 52–58.

Harrington. 1997. Post-adolescent acne and marital break-up. *Br J Dermatol* 137 (3): 478–79.

Hayashi et al. 2001. An epidemiological study of acne vulgaris in Japan by questionnaire. *Jpn J Dermatol* 111 (9): 1347–55.

Heald et al. 2003. The influence of dietary intake on the insulin-like growth factor (IGF) system across three ethnic groups: A population-based study. *Public Health Nutr* 6: 175–80.

Heaney et al. 1999. Dietary changes favorably affect bone remodeling in older adults. *J Am Diet Assoc* 99 (10): 1228–33.

Hebert et al. 2005. Physiological stress response to video-game playing: The contribution of built-in music. *Life Sci* 76 (20): 2371–80.

Heinrich et al. 2006. Long-term ingestion of high flavanol cocoa provides photoprotection against UV-induced erythema and improves skin condition in women. *J Nutr* 136 (6): 1565–69.

Hibbeln et al. 2006. Omega-3 fatty acid deficiencies in neurodevelopment, aggression and autonomic dysregulation: Opportunities for intervention. *Int Rev Psychiatry* 18 (2): 107–18.

Hill et al. 2006. The heart-mind connection. *Behav Health* 26 (9): 30–32.

Hitch and Greenburg. 1961. Adolescent acne and dietary iodine. *Arch Dermatol* 84 (December): 898–911.

Holmes et al. 2002. Dietary correlates of plasma insulin-like growth factor I and insulin-like growth factor binding protein 3 concentrations. *Cancer Epidemiol Biomarkers Prev* 11: 852–61.

Hoppe et al. 2005. High intakes of milk, but not meat, increase s-insulin and insulin resistance in 8-year-old boys. *Eur J Clin Nutr* 59 (3): 393–98.

Horrobin and Cunnane. 1979. Zinc, essential fatty acids, and prostaglandins. *Arch Dermatol* 115 (5): 641–42.

Hosoda. 1992. The gastrointestinal tract and nutrition in the aging process: An overview. *Nutr Rev* 50 (12): 372–73.

Hughes et al. 1983. Treatment of acne vulgaris by biofeedback relaxation and cognitive imagery. *J Psychosom Res* 27 (3): 185–91.

Hvas et al. 2004. Vitamin B6 level is associated with symptoms of depression. *Psychother Psychosom* 73 (6): 340–43.

Inoue et al. 2003. Autonomic nervous responses according to preference for the odor of jasmine tea. *Biosci Biotechnol Biochem* 67 (6): 1206–14.

Ivandic et al. 2002. Insulin resistance and androgens in healthy women with different body fat distributions. *Wien Klin Wochenschr* 114 (8–9): 321–26.

Iwama. 2004. Negative air ions created by water shearing improve erythrocyte deformability and aerobic metabolism. *Indoor Air* 14 (4): 293–97.

Jablonska. 1975. Treatment of acne vulgaris and rosacea. *Arch Dermatol* 111 (7): 929.

Jenkins et al. 2006. Almonds decrease postprandial glycemia, insulinemia, and oxidative damage in healthy individuals. *J Nutr* 136 (12): 2987–92.

Jolad et al. 2005. Commercially processed dry ginger (Zingiber officinale): Composition and effects on LPS-stimulated PGE2 production. *Phytochemistry* 66 (13): 1614–35.

Kagawa. 1978. Impact of Westernization on the nutrition of Japanese: Changes in physique, cancer, longevity and centenarians. *Prev Med* 7 (2): 205–17.

Kaklamani et al. 1999. Dietary fat and carbohydrates are independently associated with circulating insulin-like growth factor 1 and insulin-like growth factor-binding protein 3 concentrations in healthy adults. *J Clin Oncol* 17: 3291–98.

Kang et al. 2006. The effects of dairy processes and storage on insulin-like growth factor-I (IGF-I) content in milk and in model IGF-I-fortified dairy products. *J Dairy Sci* 89 (2): 402–9.

Kankaanpaa et al. 2002. Influence of probiotic supplemented infant formula on composition of plasma lipids in atopic infants. *J Nutr Biochem* 13 (6): 364–69.

Kankaanpaa et al. 2004. Effects of polyunsaturated fatty acids in growth medium on lipid composition and on physicochemical surface properties of lactobacilli. *Appl Environ Microbiol* 70 (1): 129–36.

Kant et al. 2003. Reported consumption of low-nutrient-density foods by American children and adolescents: Nutritional and health correlates, NHANES III, 1988 to 1994. *Arch Pediatr Adolesc Med* 157 (8): 789–96.

Kaufman. 1965. Management of acne vulgaris. *Med Times* 93: 805–12.

Kaufman. 1983. The diet and acne. *Arch Dermatol* 119 (4): 276.

Kellett and Gawkroger. 1999. The psychological and emotional impact of acne and the effect of treatment with isotretinoin. *Br J Dermatol* 140 (2): 273–82.

Khalif et al. 2005. Alterations in the colonic flora and intestinal permeability and evidence of immune activation in chronic constipation. *Dig Liver Dis* 37 (11): 838–49.

Khan et al. 2003. Cinnamon improves glucose and lipids of people with type 2 diabetes. *Diabetes Care* 26 (12): 3215–18.

Kimura et al. 2007. L-theanine reduces psychological and physiological stress responses. *Biol Psychol* 74 (1): 39–45.

King et al. 2003. Relation of dietary fat and fiber to elevation of C-reactive protein. *Am J Cardiol* 92 (11): 1335–39.

King et al. 2005. Association of stress, hostility, and plasma testosertone levels. *Nueroendocrinol Lett* 26: 355–60.

King et al. 2005. Dietary magnesium and C-reactive protein levels. *J Am Coll Nutr* 24 (3): 166–71.

Kligman. 2002. Origin of the annual symposium on the biology of skin. *J Investig Dermatol Symp Pro* 7 (1): 1–3.

Kligman et al. 1981. Oral vitamin A in acne vulgaris. Preliminary report. *Int J Dermatol* 20 (4): 278–85.

Kobasa et al. 1982. Personality and exercise as buffers in the stress-illness relationship. *J Behav Med* 5 (4): 391–404.

Koebnick et al. 2003. Probiotic beverage containing Lactobacillus casei Shirota improves gastrointestinal symptoms in patients with chronic constipation. *Can J Gastroenterol* 17 (11): 655–59.

Kolpin et al. 2002. Pharmaceuticals, hormones, and other organic wastewater contaminants in U.S. streams, 1999–2000: A national reconnaissance. *Environ Sci Technol* 36 (6): 1202–11.

Kouvonen et al. 2005. Job strain and leisure-time physical activity in female and male public sector employees. *Prev Med* 41 (2): 532–39.

Kovalev and Bensemman. 1983. Evaluation of the results of a study of prostaglandin E, E2, F and cyclic 3',5'-adenosine monophosphate content of the blood and skin homogenates of acne patients. *Vestn Dermatol Venerol* (2): 17–20.

Kovalev. 1981. Complex treatment of acne with lipoic acid. *Vrach Delo* (3): 108–13.

Kovalev. 1981. Lipoic acid content in the blood and urine in acne and its use in the treatment of this disease. *Vestn Dermatol Venerol* (3): 65–67.

Kovalev. 1982. Dynamics of the blood level of prostaglandin E2 in patients with acne undergoing combination therapy. *Vestn Dermatol Venerol* (7): 24–27.

Krejci-Manwaring et al. 2006. Social sensitivity and acne: The role of personality in negative social consequences and quality of life. *Int J Psychiatry Med* 36 (1): 121–30.

Kuda et al. 2000. Cecal environment and TBARS level in mice fed corn oil, beef tallow and menhaden fish oil. *J Nutr Sci Vitaminol* (Tokyo) 46 (2): 65–70.

Kull. 2002. The relationships between physical activity, health status and psychological well-being of fertility-aged women. *Scand J Med Sci Sports* 12 (4): 241–47.

Kunstmann and Christiansen. 2004. Testosterone levels and stress in women: The role of stress coping strategies, anxiety and sex role identification. *Anthropol Anz* 62 (3): 311–21.

Kuo and Taylor. 2004. A potential natural treatment for attention-deficit/hyperactivity disorder: Evidence from a national study. *Am J Public Health* 94 (9): 1580–86.

Kurutas et al. 2005. Superoxide dismutase and. myeloperoxidase activities in polymorphonuclear leukocytes in acne vulgaris. *Acta Dermatoven APA* 14 (2): 39–42.

Labadarios et al. 1987. Vitamin A in acne vulgaris. *Clin Exp Dermatol* 12 (6): 432–36.

Lai and Good. 2005. Music improves sleep quality in older adults. *J Adv Nurs* 49 (3): 234–44.

Lanou et al. 2005. Calcium, dairy products, and bone health in children and young adults: A reevaluation of the evidence. *Pediatrics* 115 (3): 736–43.

Lantz et al. 2005. The effect of turmeric extracts on inflammatory mediator production. *Phytomedicine* 12 (6–7): 445–52.

Lee. 2005. The effect of lavender aromatherapy on cognitive function, emotion, and aggressive behavior of elderly with dementia. *Taehan Kanho Hakhoe Chi* 35 (2): 303–12.

Lee and Lee. 2006. Effects of lavender aromatherapy on insomnia and depression in women college students. *Taehan Kanho Hakhoe Chi* 36 (1): 136–43.

Lee et al. 2006. Effect of tea phenolics and their aromatic fecal bacterial metabolites on intestinal microbiota. *Res Microbiol* 157 (9): 876–84.

Leichsenring et al. 2006. Cognitive-behavioral therapy and psychodynamic psychotherapy: Techniques, efficacy, and indications. *Am J Psychother* 60 (3): 233–59.

Leitner et al. 2005. Do the effects of job stressors on health persist over time? A longitudinal study with observational stressor measures. *J Occup Health Psychol* 10 (1): 18–30.

Leuchter et al. 2002. Changes in brain function of depressed subjects during treatment with placebo. *Am J Psychiatry* 159 (1): 122–29.

Liang and Liao. 1992. Inhibition of steroid 5 alpha-reductase by specific aliphatic unsaturated fatty acids. *Biochem J* 285 (July; pt. 2): 557–62.

Liao et al. 1995. Selective inhibition of steroid 5 alpha-reductase isozymes by tea epicatechin-3-gallate and epigallocatechin-3-gallate. *Biochem Biophys Res Commun* 214 (3): 833–38.

Lichtenthaler et al. 2005. Total oxidant scavenging capacities of Euterpe oleracea Mart. (Acai) fruits. *Int J Food Sci Nutr* 56 (1): 53–64.

Liljeberg et al. 2001. Milk as a supplement to mixed meals may elevate postprandial insulinaemia. *Eur J Clin Nutr* 55 (11): 994–99.

Livesey et al. 2005. Low-glycaemic diets and health: implications for obesity. *Proc Nutr Soc* 64 (1): 105–13.

Logan. 2003. Omega-3 fatty acids and acne. *Arch Dermatol* 139 (7): 941–42.

Lorenz et al. 1953. The relation of life stress and emotions to human sebum secretion and to the mechanism of acne vulgaris. *J Lab Clin Med* 41 (1): 11–28.

Lyons. 2002. Psychosocial factors related to job stress and women in management. *Work* 18 (1): 89–93.

Mackie and Mackie. 1974. Chocolate and acne. *Australas J Dermatol* 15 (3): 103–9.

Magin et al. 2006. Complementary and alternative medicine therapies in acne, psoriasis, and atopic eczema: Results of a qualitative study of patients' experiences and perceptions. *J Altern Complement Med* 12 (5): 451–57.

Makowske and Feinman. 2005. Nutrition education: A questionnaire for assessment and teaching. *Nutr J* 4 (January): 2.

Mallon et al. 1999. The quality of life in acne: A comparison with general medical conditions using generic questionnaires. *Br J Dermatol* 140 (4): 672–76.

Mang et al. 2006. Effects of a cinnamon extract on plasma glucose, HbA, and serum lipids in diabetes mellitus type 2. *Eur J Clin Invest* 36 (5): 340–44.

Manger and Motta. 2005. The impact of an exercise program on posttraumatic stress disorder, anxiety, and depression. *Int J Emerg Ment Health* 7 (1): 49–57.

Marangoni et al. 2006. Levels of the n-3 fatty acid eicosapentaenoic acid in addition to those of alpha linolenic acid are significantly raised in blood lipids by the intake of four walnuts a day in humans. *Nutr Metab Cardiovasc Dis* (September) [Epub ahead of print].

Marchetti et al. 1987. Efficacy of regulators of the intestinal bacterial flora in the therapy of acne vulgaris. *Clin Ter* 122 (5): 339–43.

Margolis et al. 2005. Antibiotic treatment of acne may be associated with upper respiratory tract infections. *Arch Dermatol* 141 (9): 1132–36.

Mariman. 2006. Nutrigenomics and nutrigenetics: The "omics" revolution in nutritional science. *Biotechnol Appl Biochem* 44 (June; pt. 3): 119–28.

Markus et al. 2000. Effects of food on cortisol and mood in vulnerable subjects under controllable and uncontrollable stress. *Physiol Behav* 70 (3–4): 333–42.

Masuda et al. 2004. Repeated sauna therapy reduces urinary 8-epi-prostaglandin F(2alpha). *Jpn Heart J* 45 (2): 297–303.

Masuda et al. 2005. The effects of repeated thermal therapy for patients with chronic pain. *Psychother Psychosom* 74 (5): 288–94.

Maurer et al. 2003. Neutralization of Western diet inhibits bone resorption independently of K intake and reduces cortisol secretion in humans. *Am J Physiol Renal Physiol* 284 (1): F32–40.

Maxwell et al. 2002. Antibiotics increase functional abdominal symptoms. *Am J Gastroenterol* 97 (1): 104–8.

McCann et al. 1990. Changes in plasma lipids and dietary intake accompanying shifts in perceived workload and stress. *Psychosom Med* 52 (1): 97–108.

McCarty. 1984. High-chromium yeast for acne? *Med Hypotheses* 14 (3): 307–10.

McCarty et al. 1998. The effects of different types of music on mood, tension, and mental clarity. *Altern Ther Health Med* 4 (1): 75–84.

McIntyre et al. 1968. Cutaneous extracellular glucose kinetics in acne patients receiving phenformin. *Ann N Y Acad Sci* 148 (3): 833–39.

McLean. 2005. Do substance P and the NK1 receptor have a role in depression and anxiety? *Curr Pharm Des* 11 (12): 1529–47.

Messina et al. 2003. A new food guide for North American vegetarians. *Can J Diet Pract Res* 64 (2): 82–86.

Messina et al. 2006. Estimated Asian adult soy protein and isoflavone intakes. *Nutr Cancer* 55 (1): 1–12.

Michaelsson. 1990. Decreased concentration of selenium in whole blood and plasma in acne vulgaris. *Acta Derm Venereol* 70 (1): 92.

Michaelsson and Edqvist. 1984. Erythrocyte glutathione peroxidase activity in acne vulgaris and the effect of selenium and vitamin E treatment. *Acta Derm Venereol* 64 (1): 9–14.

Michaelsson and Ljunghall. 1990. Patients with dermatitis herpetiformis, acne, psoriasis and Darier's disease have low epidermal zinc concentrations. *Acta Derm Venereol* 70 (4): 304–8.

Michaelsson et al. 1977. Effects of oral zinc and vitamin A in acne. *Arch Dermatol* 113 (1): 31–36.

Michalsen et al. 2005. Rapid stress reduction and anxiolysis among distressed women as a consequence of a three-month intensive yoga program. *Med Sci Monit* 11 (12): CR555–61.

Michelson et al. 2000. Hormonal markers of stress response following interruption of selective serotonin reuptake inhibitor treatment. *Psychoneuroendocrinology* 25 (2): 169–77.

Molinski and Rechenberger. 1977. Psychosomatics of acne. *Fortschr Med* 95 (25): 2149–53.

Montrose and Floch. 2005. Probiotics used in human studies. *J Clin Gastroenterol* 39 (6): 469–84.

Moran et al. 1999. Insulin resistance during puberty: results from clamp studies in 357 children. *Diabetes* 48 (10): 2039–44.

Mori. 2004. Effect of fish and fish oil-derived omega-3 fatty acids on lipid oxidation. *Redox Rep* 9 (4): 193–97.

Morita et al. 2006. Psychological effects of forest environments on healthy adults: Shinrin-yoku (forest-air bathing, walking) as a possible method of stress reduction. *Public Health* (October) [Epub ahead of print].

Moss et al. 2003. Aromas of rosemary and lavender essential oils differentially affect cognition and mood in healthy adults. *Int J Neurosci* 113 (1): 15–38.

Mozaffarian and Rimm. 2006. Fish intake, contaminants, and human health: Evaluating the risks and the benefits. *JAMA* 296 (15): 1885–99.

Murata. 2000. Secular trends in growth and changes in eating patterns of Japanese children. *Am J Clin Nutr* 72 (5 Suppl): 1379S–1383S.

Nagata et al. 2000. Inverse association of soy product intake with serum androgen and estrogen concentrations in Japanese men. *Nutr Cancer* 36 (1): 14–18.

Nagata et al. 2000. Relationships between types of fat consumed and serum estrogen and androgen concentrations in Japanese men. *Nutr Cancer* 38 (2): 163–67.

Nakamura et al. 2000. Determination of the levels of isoflavonoids in soybeans and soy-derived foods and estimation of isoflavonoids in the Japanese daily intake. *J AOAC Int* 83 (3): 635–50.

Nakane et al. 2002. Effect of negative air ions on computer operation, anxiety and salivary chromogranin A-like immunoreactivity. *Int J Psychophysiol* 46 (1): 85–89.

Naruszewicz et al. 2002. Effect of Lactobacillus plantarum 299v on cardiovascular disease risk factors in smokers. *Am J Clin Nutr* 76 (6): 1249–55.

Nathan et al. 2006. The neuropharmacology of L-theanine(N-ethyl-L-glutamine): A possible neuroprotective and cognitive enhancing agent. *J Herb Pharmacother* 6 (2): 21–30.

Neukman et al. 2006. Consumption of flavanol-rich cocoa acutely increases micro-circulation in human skin. *Eur J Nutr* (December) [Epub ahead of print].

Newman et al. 2007. Daily hassles and eating behavior: The role of cortisol reactivity status. *Psychoneuroendocrinology* 32 (2): 125–32.

Ngo et al. 2002. Effect of diet and exercise on serum insulin, IGF-I, and IGFBP-1 levels and growth of LNCaP cells in vitro (United States). *Cancer Causes Control* 13 (10): 929–35.

Niren and Torok. 2006. The Nicomide Improvement in Clinical Outcomes Study (NICOS): Results of an 8-week trial. *Cutis* 77 (1 Suppl): 17–28.

Norrish and Dwyer. 2005. Preliminary investigation of the effect of peppermint oil on an objective measure of daytime sleepiness. *Int J Psychophysiol* 55 (3): 291–98.

Noverr et al. 2004. Role of antibiotics and fungal microbiota in driving pulmonary allergic responses. *Infect Immun* 72 (9): 4996–5003.

Nowak et al. 2005. Zinc and depression: An update. *Pharmacol Rep* 57 (6): 713–18.

Nunez et al. 2002. Effects of psychological stress and alprazolam on development of oral candidiasis in rats. *Clin Diagn Lab Immunol* 9 (4): 852–57.

Oh et al. 2006. Effect of bacteriocin produced by Lactococcus sp. HY 449 on skin-inflammatory bacteria. *Food Chem Toxicol* 44 (8): 1184–90.

Ohara K. 1969. The present status of the treatment of acne vulgaris in Japan. *J Am Med Womens Assoc* 24 (4): 313–18.

Ohtsuka et al. 1998. Shinrin-yoku (forest-air bathing and walking) effectively decreases blood glucose levels in diabetic patients. *Int J Biometeorol* 41 (3): 125–27.

O'Reilly et al. 2006. Chronic administration of 13-cis-retinoic acid increases depression-related behavior in mice. *Neuropsychopharmacology* 31 (9): 1919–27.

Ostman et al. 2001. Inconsistency between glycemic and insulinemic responses to regular and fermented milk products. *Am J Clin Nutr* 74 (1): 96–100.

Ouwehand et al. 2003. Probiotics for the skin: A new area of potential application? *Lett Appl Microbiol* 36 (5): 327–31.

Oxman et al. 2001. Oral administration of Lactobacillus induces cardioprotection. *J Altern Complement Med* 7 (4): 345–54.

Pajonk et al. 2006. The effects of tea extracts on proinflammatory signaling. *BMC Med* 4 (December): 28.

Pandey et al. 1980. Has acne urban bias? *Indian J Derm Venereol Leprol* 46 (2): 80–82.

Paraskevaidis et al. 1998. Polymorphisms in the human cytochrome P-450 1A1 gene (CYP1A1) as a factor for developing acne. *Dermatology* 196 (1): 171–75.

Penedo and Dahn. 2005. Exercise and well-being: A review of mental and physical health benefits associated with physical activity. *Curr Opin Psychiatry* 18 (2): 189–93.

Pennebaker. 1999. The effects of traumatic disclosure on physical and mental health: The values of writing and talking about upsetting events. *Int J Emerg Ment Health* 1 (1): 9–18.

Penson et al. 2005. Laughter: The best medicine? *Oncologist* 10: 651–60.

Perseghin et al. 2001. Gender factors affect fatty acids-induced insulin resistance in nonobese humans: Effects of oral steroidal contraception. *J Clin Endocrinol Metab* 86 (7): 3188–96.

Potau et al. 1997. Pubertal changes in insulin secretion and peripheral insulin sensitivity. *Horm Res* 48 (5): 219–26.

Prior and Wu. 2006. Anthocyanins: Structural characteristics that result in unique metabolic patterns and biological activities. *Free Radic Res* 40 (10): 1014–28.

Probart et al. 2005. Competitive foods available in Pennsylvania public high schools. *J Am Diet Assoc* 105 (8): 1243–49.

Probst-Hensch et al. 2003. Determinants of circulating insulin-like growth factor I and insulin-like growth factor binding protein 3 concentrations in a cohort of Singapore men and women. *Cancer Epidemiol Biomarkers Prev* 12: 739–46.

Purvis et al. 2006. Acne, anxiety, depression and suicide in teenagers: A cross-sectional survey of New Zealand secondary school students. *J Paediatr Child Health* 42 (12): 793–96.

Quinkler et al. 2004. Androgen generation in adipose tissue in women with simple obesity: A site-specific role for 17beta-hydroxysteroid dehydrogenase type 5. *J Endocrinol* 183 (2): 331–42.

Rapp et al. 2004. Anger and acne: Implications for quality of life, patient satisfaction and clinical care. *Br J Dermatol* 151 (1): 183–89.

Rasmussen. 1977. Diet and acne. *Int J Dermatol* 16 (6): 488–92.

Reich et al. 2007. Acne vulgaris: What teenagers think about it. *Dermatol Nurs* 19 (1): 49–54, 64.

Robinson HM. 1949. The acne problem. *South Med J* 42 (12): 1050–60.

Rosenberg and Kirk. 1981. Acne diet reconsidered. *Arch Dermatol* 117 (4): 193–95.

Ross. 2005. Optical treatments for acne. *Dermatol Ther* 18 (3): 253–66.

Saeki et al. 2000. The effect of foot-bath with or without the essential oil of lavender on the autonomic nervous system: A randomized trial. *Complement Ther Med* 8 (1): 2–7.

Sahud et al. 2007. The effect of a high-protein, low glycemic-load diet versus a conventional, high glycemic-load diet on biochemical parameters associated with acne vulgaris: A randomized, investigator-masked, controlled trial. *J Am Acad Dermatol* (April 18) [Epub ahead of print].

Salvador et al. 2003. Anticipatory cortisol, testosterone and psychological responses to judo competition in young men. *Psychoneuroendocrinology* 28 (3): 364–75.

Sapolsky. 2004. *Why Zebras Don't Get Ulcers.* New York: Owl Books/Henry Holt and Co.

Sasaki et al. 2003. Self-reported rate of eating correlates with body mass index in 18-year-old Japanese women. *Int J Obes Relat Metab Disord* 27 (11): 1405–10.

Savino et al. 2007. Lactobacillus reuteri (American Type Culture Collection Strain 55730) versus simethicone in the treatment of infantile colic: A prospective randomized study. *Pediatrics* 119 (1): e124–30.

Schaefer. 1971. When the Eskimo comes to town. *Nutr Today* 6: 8–16.

Schafer et al. 2001. Epidemiology of acne in the general population: The risk of smoking. *Br J Dermatol* 145 (1): 100–104.

Schaffer. 1989. Essential fatty acids and eicosanoids in cutaneous inflammation. *Int J Dermatol* 28 (5): 281–90.

Schmidt et al. 1990. Endocrine parameters in acne vulgaris. *Endocrinol Exp* 24 (4): 457–64.

Schulman JA. 1999. Nutrition education in medical schools: Trends and implications for health educators. *Med Educ Online* 4: http://www.med-edonline.org.

Schulpis et al. 2001. Elevated plasma homocysteine levels in patients on isotretinoin therapy for cystic acne. *Int J Dermatol* 40 (1): 33–36.

Scott-Kantor. 1996. Many Americans are not meeting food guide pyramid dietary recommendations—includes related articles on recommended serving and on food supply series—Moving Toward Healthier Diets. *Food Review* (January–February).

Shalita et al. 1995. Topical nicotinamide compared with clindamycin gel in the treatment of inflammatory acne vulgaris. *Int J Dermatol* 34 (6): 434–37.

Shaw. 2001. Green tea polyphenols may be useful in the treatment of androgen-mediated skin disorders. *Arch Dermatol* 137 (5): 664.

Sheu et al. 1994. Prospective evaluation of insulin resistance and lipid metabolism in women receiving oral contraceptives. *Clin Endocrinol* (Oxf) 40 (2): 249–55.

Silverberg and Weinberg. 2001. Rosacea and adult acne: A worldwide epidemic. *Cutis* 68 (2): 85.

Simopoulos. 2001. The Mediterranean diets: What is so special about the diet of Greece? The scientific evidence. *J Nutr* 131 (11 Suppl): 3065S–3073S.

Simopoulos et al. 1999. Workshop on the essentiality of and recommended dietary intakes for omega-6 and omega-3 fatty acids. *J Am Coll Nutr* 18 (5): 487–89.

Siver. 1961. Lactobacillus for the control of acne. *J Med Soc New Jersey* 59 (2): 52–53.

Skidmore et al. 2003. Effects of subantimicrobial-dose doxycycline in the treatment of moderate acne. *Arch Dermatol* 139 (4): 459–64.

Sluzberger and Zaidems. 1948. Psychogenic factors in dermatological disorders. *Medical Clinics of North America* 32: 669–73.

Smith. 2002. Stress, breakfast cereal consumption and cortisol. *Nutr Neurosci* 5 (2): 141–44.

Smith et al. 2001. High fiber breakfast cereals reduce fatigue. *Appetite* 37 (3): 249–50.

Smith et al. 2003. Cutaneous expression of cytochrome P450 CYP2S1: Individuality in regulation by therapeutic agents for psoriasis and other skin diseases. *Lancet* 361 (9366): 1336–43.

Smith et al. 2005. Low glycemic load, high protein diet lessens facial acne severity. *Asia Pac J Clin Nutr* 14 (Suppl): S97.

Smith et al. 2006. Insulin-like growth factor-1 induces lipid production in human SEB-1 sebocytes via sterol response element-binding protein-1. *J Invest Dermatol* 126 (6): 1226–32.

Solberg et al. 2004. The effects of long meditation on plasma melatonin and blood serotonin. *Med Sci Monit* 10 (3): CR96–101.

Songisepp et al. 2005. Evaluation of the functional efficacy of an antioxidative probiotic in healthy volunteers. *Nutr J* 4 (August): 22.

Sorg et al. 2007. Effect of intense pulsed-light exposure on lipid peroxides and thymine dimers in human skin in vivo. *Arch Dermatol* 143 (3): 363–66.

Spencer et al. 2006. Predictors of nutrition counseling behaviors and attitudes in US medical students. *Am J Clin Nutr* 84 (3): 655–62.

Steptoe and Wardle. 1998. Stress, hassles and variations in alcohol consumption, food choice and physical exercise: A diary study. *Br J Health Psych* 3: 51–63.

Stolberg. Superbugs. *New York Times*, August 2, 1998.

Strauss et al. 1967. Suppression of sebaceous gland activity with eicosa-5:8:11:14-tetraynoic acid. *J Invest Dermatol* 48 (5): 492–93.

Strohle et al. 2005. The acute antipanic activity of aerobic exercise. *Am J Psychiatry* 162 (12): 2376–78.

Sundquist et al. 2004. Urbanization and incidence of psychosis and depression: Follow-up study of 4.4 million women and men in Sweden. *Br J Psychiatry* 184 (April): 293–98.

Surette et al. 2003. Inhibition of leukotriene synthesis, pharmacokinetics, and tolerability of a novel dietary fatty acid formulation in healthy adult subjects. *Clin Ther* 25 (3): 948–71.

Svartberg and Jorde. 2006. Endogenous testosterone levels and smoking in men. The fifth Tromso study. *Int J Androl* (November) [Epub ahead of print].

Takatsuka et al. 2000. Changes in microbial flora in neutropenic patients with hematological disorders after the Hanshin-Awaji earthquake. *Int J Hematol* 71 (3): 273–77.

Takeda et al. 2004. Stress control and human nutrition. *J Med Invest* 51 (3–4): 139–45.

Templeton et al. 2005. Competitive foods increase the intake of energy and decrease the intake of certain nutrients by adolescents consuming school lunch. *J Am Diet Assoc* 105 (2): 215–20.

Ten Bruggencate et al. 2005. Dietary fructooligosaccharides increase intestinal permeability in rats. *J Nutr* 135 (4): 837–42.

Ten Bruggencate et al. 2006. Dietary fructooligosaccharides affect intestinal barrier function in healthy men. *J Nutr* 136 (1): 70–74.

Tomei et al. 2004. Occupational exposure to urban pollutants and plasma insulin-like growth factor 1 (IGF-1). *Int J Environ Health Res* 14 (2): 135–42.

Torok. 2006. Nicotinamide and zinc in the treatment of acne and rosacea. *Cutis* 77 (1 Suppl): 3–4.

Toyoda and Morohashi. 2003. New aspects in acne inflammation. *Dermatology* 206 (1): 17–23.

Tsai et al. 2006. Higher body mass index is a significant risk factor for acne formation in schoolchildren. *Eur J Dermatol* 16 (3): 251–53.

Uhe et al. 1992. A comparison of the effects of beef, chicken and fish protein on satiety and amino acid profiles in lean male subjects. *J Nutr* 122 (3): 467–72.

Unger et al. 2004. Acculturation, physical activity, and fast-food consumption among Asian-American and Hispanic adolescents. *J Community Health* 29 (6): 467–81.

Velicer et al. 2004. Antibiotic use in relation to the risk of breast cancer. *JAMA* 291 (7): 827–35.

Verhulst et al. 1987. Isomerization of polyunsaturated long chain fatty acids by Propionobacteria. *Syst Appl Microbiol* 9: 12–15.

Vierhapper and Nowotny. 2000. The stress of being a doctor: Steroid excretion rates in internal medicine residents on and off duty. *Am J Med* 109 (6): 492–94.

Vignes et al. 2006. Anxiolytic properties of green tea polyphenol (-)-epigallocatechin gallate (EGCG). *Brain Res* 1110 (1): 102–15.

Viladiu et al. 1996. A breast cancer case-control study in Girona, Spain. Endocrine, familial and lifestyle factors. *Eur J Cancer Prev* 5 (5): 329–35.

Vlassara. 2005. Advanced glycation in health and disease: Role of the modern environment. *Ann N Y Acad Sci* 1043 (June): 452–60.

Volkova et al. 2001. Impact of the impaired intestinal microflora on the course of acne vulgaris. *Klin Med* (Mosk) 79 (6): 39–41.

Wang and Wu. 2005. Effects of psychological stress on small intestinal motility and bacteria and mucosa in mice. *World J Gastroenterol* 11 (13): 2016–21.

Wang et al. 2005. Low-fat high-fiber diet decreased serum and urine androgens in men. *J Clin Endocrinol Metab* 90 (6): 3550–59.

Watanabe et al. 2006. Differences in relaxation by means of guided imagery in a healthy community sample. *Altern Ther Health Med* 12 (2): 60–66.

Weiss and Anderton. 2003. Determination of catechins in matcha green tea by micellar electrokinetic chromatography. *J Chromatogr A* 1011 (1–2): 173–80.

West et al. 2004. Effects of Hatha yoga and African dance on perceived stress, affect, and salivary cortisol. *Ann Behav Med* 28 (2): 114–18.

Wilson et al. 2005. Characteristics of pediatric and adolescent patients attending a naturopathic college clinic in Canada. *Pediatrics* 115 (3): e338–43.

Winick. 1993. Nutrition education in medical schools. *Am J Clin Nutr* 58 (6): 825–27.

Woo-Sam. 1979. The effect of vitamin A acid on experimentally induced comedone: an electron microscope study. *Br J Dermatol* 100 (3): 267–76.

Wu et al. 2004. Lipophilic and hydrophilic antioxidant capacities of common foods in the United States. *J Agric Food Chem* 52 (12): 4026–37.

Wyatt et al. 2006. Overweight and obesity: Prevalence, consequences, and causes of a growing public health problem. *Am J Med Sci* 331 (4): 166–74.

Yamaguchi et al. 2006. The effects of exercise in forest and urban environments on sympathetic nervous activity of normal young adults. *J Int Med Res* 34 (2): 152–59.

Zanarini and Frankenburg. 2003. Omega-3 fatty acid treatment of women with borderline personality disorder: A double-blind, placebo-controlled pilot study. *Am J Psychiatry* 160 (1): 167–69.

Zhang et al. 2005. How does a suicide attempter eat differently from others? Comparison of macronutrient intakes. *Nutrition* 21 (6): 711–17.

Zouboulis. 2005. Sebaceous glands and the prostaglandin pathway: Key stones of an exciting mosaic. *J Invest Dermatol* 125 (5): x–xi.

Zouboulis et al. 2003. A new concept for acne therapy: A pilot study with zileuton, an oral 5-lipoxygenase inhibitor. *Arch Dermatol* 139 (5): 668–70.

Zouboulis et al. 2005. Zileuton, an oral 5-lipoxygenase inhibitor, directly reduces sebum production. *Dermatology* 210 (1): 36–38.

Appendix

RESOURCES

More on Dr. Valori Treloar, including information on integrative dermatology and printable Clear Skin resources: www.integrativederm.com.

More on Dr. Alan C. Logan, including additional articles, foods and recommended dietary supplements: www.drlogan.com.

FURTHER READING

Omnivore's Dilemma. Michael Pollan (Penguin Press, 2006).

The Relaxation Response. Herbert Benson and Miriam Klipper (Harper, 2000).

Why Zebras Don't Get Ulcers. Robert Sapolsky (Owl Books, 2004).

Eat, Drink and Be Healthy. Walter Willet (Free Press, 2005).

The End of Stress As We Know It. Bruce McEwen and Elizabeth Lasley (Dana Press, 2004).

Ultraprevention. Mark Hyman and Mark Liponis (Atris, 2005).

The Schwarzbein Principle. Diana Schwarzbein and Nancy Deville (HCI, 1999).

The Food Connection. Sam Graci (Wiley, 2006).

HAND-HELD THERMAL ANTIACNE THERAPY

The Zeno
  Tyrell Inc.
  515 W. Greens Rd., Suite 725
  Houston, TX 77067
  www.myzeno.com

SKIN-CARE PRODUCTS

Neutrogena Fresh Foaming Cleanser
  Neutrogena Corporation
  5760 W. 96th St.
  Los Angeles, CA 90045
  (800) 421-6857
  www.neutrogena.com

Cetaphil Cleanser for Normal and Oily Skin
Galderma Laboratories
14501 N. Freeway
Ft. Worth, TX 76177
(817) 961-5000
www.cetaphil.com

Dermalogica clearing skin wash & anti-bacterial skin wash
Dermalogica
1535 Beachey Place
Carson, CA 90746
(310) 900-4000
www.dermalogica.com
Includes natural botanicals and no artificial colors or fragrances

ANXIETY AND STRESS

Anxiety and Phobia Treatment Center at White Plains Hospital
Support Groups and Anxiety/Stress Management Courses
Davis Ave. at East Post Rd.
White Plains, NY 10601
(914) 681-1038
www.phobia-anxiety.org

The American Institute of Stress
124 Park Ave.
Yonkers, NY 10703
(914) 963-1200
www.stress.org

Harvard Mind-Body Medical Institute Programs
824 Boylston St.
Chestnut Hill, MA 02467
(617) 991-0102
(866) 509-0732
www.mbmi.org

The Center for Mind-Body Medicine
5225 Connecticut Ave, NW
Suite 414
Washington, DC 20015
(202) 966-7338
www.cmbm.org

NUTRITIONALLY ORIENTED MEDICAL DOCTORS AND NATUROPATHIC PHYSICIANS

American Holistic Medical Association
12101 Menaul Blvd., NE, Suite C
Albuquerque, NM 87112
(505) 292-7788
(505) 293-7582
www.holisticmedicine.org

The American Association of Naturopathic Physicians
    3201 New Mexico Avenue, NW Suite 350
    Washington, DC 20016
    (866) 538-2267
    (202) 895-1392
    Fax: (202) 274-1992
    www.naturopathic.org
Canadian Association of Naturopathic Doctors
    1255 Sheppard Ave. E., Toronto
    Canada M2K1E2
    (416) 496-8633
    (800) 551-4381
    Fax: (416) 496-8634
    www.naturopathicassoc.ca

NUTRITION CONTINUING MEDICAL EDUCATION FOR HEALTHCARE PROVIDERS

Food as Medicine
    Sponsored by Georgetown University School of Medicine
    www.cmbm.org
The Institute for Functional Medicine
    Annual symposium approved by the Accreditation Council for Continuing
    Medical Education
    www.functionalmedicine.org

ENVIRONMENTAL AND NUTRITIONAL CONTAMINANTS

The Environmental Working Group
    1436 U Street NW, Suite 100
    Washington, DC 20009
    (202) 667-6982
    http://www.ewg.org
    Provides up to date information on mercury in fish, and pesticides on produce

MERCURY TESTING

Sierra Club
    85 Second Street, 2nd Floor
    San Francisco, CA 94105
    (415) 977-5500
    www.sierraclub.com/mercury

OMEGA-3 SUPPLEMENT INDEPENDENT QUALITY ASSURANCE

International Fish Oil Standards
    Nutrasource Diagnostics
    Granbry Building Suite 4
    130 Research Lane
    University of Guelph Research Park
    Guelph, Ontario, Canada
    N1G 5G3
    (877) 557-7722
    www.nutrasource.ca
    Provides public disclosure of independent testing on commercial fish oil
    supplements

NUTRITIONAL SUPPLEMENTS

Drs. Treloar and Logan are very particular when it concerns endorsing dietary supplements. Quality is non-negotiable for our patients and our own reputations. Multivitamin-mineral formulas must be free of food dyes, fillers, and other artificial ingredients. Essential fatty acids must be non-rancid and free of mercury, PCBs, and other environmental toxins.

Genuine Health Inc
   317 Adelaide St West, 501
   Toronto, ON M5V 1P9
   (416) 977-8765
   (877) 500-7888
   Perfect Skin, the concentrated, pharmaceutical-grade omega-3 EPA along with added zinc, selenium, chromium and EGCG from green tea. Genuine Health is a science-based company, and product development is based primarily on filling in the nutritional voids in North America. They are also the manufacturers of greens+ and work closely with university-based scientists and have conducted original research on products at the University of Toronto.
   www.genuinehealth.com or http://ca.genuinehealth.com

ZenBev™
   Biosential Inc.
   1543 Bayview Ave., Suite 346
   Toronto, ON M4G 3B5
   Canada
   (800) 735-4538
   (416) 421-7445
   www.zenbev.com

Metagenics, Inc.
   9770 44th Ave. N.W., Suite 100
   Gig Habor, WA 98332
   (800) 843-9660
   www.metagenics.com

Nordica Naturals
   94 Hangar Way
   Watsonville, CA 95076
   (800) 662-2544
   www.nordicnaturals.com

PROBIOTICS

Lactobacillus plantarum 299V (LactoFlamX)
   Metagenics, Inc.
   9770 44th Ave. N.W., Suite 100
   Gig Harbor, WA 98332
   (800) 843-9660
   www.metagenics.com

Lactobacillus casei strain Shirota

Yakult International (USA)
    3510 Torrance Blvd., Suite 216
    Torrance, CA 90503
    (310) 792-1422
    Contact: Hisashi Satoi
    e-mail hisashi-satoi896@yakultusa.com
    www.yakult.co.jp/english/

Lactobacillus GG

Culturelle™
    ConAgra Foods
    One ConAgra Drive
    Omaha, NE 68102
    (402) 595-4000
    (888) 828-4242
    e-mail : culturelle@conagrafoods.com
Align™ (Bifidobacterium infantis 35624)
    1 Procter & Gamble Plaza
    Cincinnati, Ohio 45202
    (800) 208-0112
    www.aligngi.com
    Highly researched probiotic proven to lower inflammatory markers outside the gut.

Biofeedback Supplies for Meditation and Mind-Body Exercises

Biodot of Indiana Inc.
    P.O. Box 2246
    Indianapolis, IN 46206
    800 367-1604
    http://www.stressstop.com

StressEraser

Helicor, Inc.
    156 5th Avenue
    Suite 1218
    New York, NY 10010
    www.stresseraser.com

Sauna

SaunaRay Home Saunas
    877 992-1100
    www.saunaray.com
    e-mail: info@saunaray.com

NEGATIVE AIR ION GENERATOR

SphereOne, Inc.
    945 Main St./P.O. Box 1013
    Silver Plume, CO 80476
    www.sphereone.com
    (800) 858-3229

HEALTH FOOD CHAINS

Whole Foods Market, Inc.
    550 Bowie St.
    Austin, TX 78703-4677
    (512) 477-4455
    Voicemail: (512) 477-5566
    Fax: (512) 482-7000
    www.wholefoodsmarket.com
Wild Oats Markets, Inc.
    3375 Mitchell Lane
    Boulder, CO 80301
    (800) 494-9453
    www.wildoats.com

JAPANESE FOODS

Mitsuwa Marketplace
    595 River Rd.
    Edgewater, NJ 07020
    (201) 941-9113
    Nine retail markets in the United States
Nippan Daido
    522 Mamaroneck Ave.
    White Plains, NY 10605
    (914) 683-6735
    Three retail markets in the United States

ON-LINE SOURCE OF JAPANESE MATCHA, GREEN TEA NOODLES, SESAME AND POLYPHENOL-RICH CHOCOLATE

www.kenkonutrition.com

NUTRITION INFORMATION AND TRADITIONAL REGIONAL DIETS

Oldways Preservation & Exchange Trust
    266 Beacon St.
    Boston, MA 02116
    (617) 421-5500
    www.oldwayspt.org
    Oldways is the widely-respected nonprofit "food issues think tank" praised for
    translating the complex details of nutrition science into "the familiar language
    of food." This synthesis converts high-level science into a consumer-friendly
    health-promotion tool for all. Jointly with the Harvard School of Public Health
    and other institutions, Oldways has published the "healthy eating pyramids," a
    set of unique dietary guides based on worldwide dietary traditions closely asso-
    ciated with good health.

Frozen Seafood Burgers—Shrimp, Tuna, Mahi-Mahi and Salmon

Omega Foods Ltd.
   P.O. Box 21256
   Eugene, OR 97402
   (541) 349-0731
   www.omegafoods.com

Organic Soup Stocks with No added Chemicals

Imagine Foods
   The Hain Celestial Group
   4600 Sleepytime Dr.
   Boulder, CO 80301
   (800) 434-4246
   www.imaginefoods.com

Healthy Snacks and Salad Dressing/Dipping Sauces with No Added Chemicals

Sahale Snacks
   P.O. Box 9345
   Seattle, WA 98109
   www.sahalesnacks.com
Mrs. May's Naturals
   12436 Bell Ranch Dr.
   Santa Fe Springs, CA 90670
   (562) 906-0345
   www.mrsmays.com
The Ginger People
   Royal Pacific Foods
   Monterey, CA 93940
   (800) 551-5284
   www.gingerpeople.com

Antioxidant Foods

Booster Juice
   4949 Meadows Rd., Suite 375
   Lake Oswego, OR 97035
   www.boosterjuice.com
International Tree Nut Council
   2413 Anza Ave.
   Davis, CA 95616
   (530) 297-5895
   www.nuthealth.org
Acai Amazon Palmberry
   SAMBAZON
   927 Calle Negocio, Suite J
   San Clemente, CA 92673
   (877) SAMBAZON
   www.sambazon.com

Wild Blueberry Association of North America
   P.O. Box 1130
   Kennebunkport, Maine 04046
   (207) 967-5024
   www.wildblueberries.com

Pomegranate Juice
   POM Wonderful, LLC
   11444 West Olympic Blvd.
   Los Angeles, CA 90064
   (310) 966-5800
   www.pomwonderful.com

Index

About the Authors

Alan C. Logan, ND, FRSH, is a board-certified naturopathic physician licensed in Connecticut. He graduated magna cum laude from the State University of New York at Purchase, and as valedictorian from the Canadian College of Naturopathic Medicine. He is an invited faculty member in Harvard's School of Continuing Medical Education where he lectures in the mind-body medicine courses. He is the only naturopathic doctor to have his commentaries published in the three leading dermatology journals—*Archives of Dermatology*, the *International Journal of Dermatology* and the *Journal of the American Academy of Dermatology*. He is author of the best-selling book *The Brain Diet* and lives in Westchester County, New York.

Valori Treloar, MD, FAAD, CNS, is a board-certified dermatologist who trained at the Boston University–Tufts University Joint Training Program in Dermatology after graduating from Boston University School of Medicine. She is the only dermatologist to earn Certified Nutritionist Specialist status from the American College of Nutrition. She is a member of the Institute for Functional Medicine and completed the course Applying Functional Medicine in Clinical Practice, offered by that organization. Val lives with her husband, daughter, and son within walking distance of her Integrative Dermatology office in Newton, Massachusetts.